i

this is a z
been sexua
answers, j

the heart of it, the hurt and fear and aloneness, the helplessness and failures and how we have pulled through, what we have learned, how we have grown, what we can teach eachother.

> we are not alone
> we are not alone

In my ideal world, people who weren't abused would talk to eachother and learn from eachother ways to support and understand us; their friends + lovers who have particularly complicated bodies and thoughts.

and us - we would not have to be so afraid to talk to eachother about ways we've survived, ways we've grown.

We'd see that growth is possible. that good communication (with ourselves + with our important ones) is something we can let ouselves want, something we can work towards + demand + even get (someday)

in my ideal world, none of us would have been abused in the first place!

the original intention of this zine was to help people who weren't abused figure out ways to be supportive, but I think a lot of the writing in here is useful for all of us.

If you have been abused, this subject could be really triggering. And we don't all have a friend we can call when we're freaking out. So, seriously, I am asking you, if you think you could be triggered in destructive ways by this, please wait. put the zine down. think of things you could do to minimize the harm you might do to yourself. Try to make your space safe and gather what inner support you have.

also, you don't have to read this right now.

If you do have a friend to call, make sure they'll be available.

here's some crisis line #s just in case: 1-800-SUICIDE
1-800-656-HOPE (sexual assault survivors hotline)

consent

One really important way to be supportive is to make sure that you, yourself, aren't doing things that may be abusive.

A few years ago, me and andrea put together this list of questions about consent. Not all of the questions have right or wrong answers. We put them together with the hopes that it would help people to think deeply, and to help open up conversations about consent.

I know it's a long list, but please read and think honestly about these question, one at a time.

1. How do you define consent?
2. Have you ever talked about consent with your partner(s) or friends
3. Do you know people, or have you been with people who define consent differently than you do?
4. Have you ever been unsure about whether or not the person you were being sexual with wanted to be doing what you were doing? Did you talk about it? Did you ignore it in hopes that it would change? Did you continue what you were doing because it was pleasurable to you and you didn't want to deal with what the other person was experiencing? Did you continue because you didn't want to second-guess the other person? Did you continue because you felt it was your duty? How do you feel about the choices you made?
5. Do you think it is the other person's responsibility to say something if they aren't into what you're doing?
6. How might someone express that what is happening is not ok?
7. Do you look only for verbal signs or are there other signs?
8. Do you think it is possible to misinterpret silence for consent?
9. Have you ever asked someone what kinds of signs you should look for if they have a hard time verbalizing when something feels wrong?
10. Do you only ask about these kinds of things if you are in a serious relationship or do you feel comfortable talking in casual situations too?
11. Do you think talking ruins the mood?
12. Do you think consent can be erotic?
13. Do you think about people's abuse histories?
14. Do you check in as things progress or do you assume the original consent means everything is ok?
15. If you achieve consent once, do you assume it's always ok after that?
16. If someone consents to one thing, do you assume everything else is ok or do you ask before touching in different ways or taking things to more intense levels?
17. Are you resentful of people who want or need to talk about being abuse? Why?
18. Are you usually attracted to people who fit the traditional standard of beauty as seen in the united states?
19. Do you pursue friendship with people because you want to be with them, and then give up on the friendship if that person isn't interested in you sexually?
20. Do you pursue someone sexually even after they have said they just want to be friends?
21. Do you assume that if someone is affectionate they are probably sexually interested in you?
22. Do you think about affection, sexuality and boundaries? Do you talk about these issues with people? If so, do you talk about them only when you want to be sexual with someone or do you talk about them because you think it is important and you genuinely want to know?

23. Are you clear about your own intentions?
24. Have you ever tried to talk someone into doing something they showed hesitancy about?
25. Do you think hesitancy is a form of flirting?
26. Are you aware that in some instances it is not?
27. Have you ever thought someone's actions were flirtatious when that wasn't actually the message they wanted to get across?
28. Do you think that if someone is promiscuous that makes it ok to objectify them, or talk about them in ways you normally wouldn't?
29. If someone is promiscuous, do you think it's less important to get consent?
30. Do you think that if someone dresses in a certain way it makes it ok to objectify them?
31. If someone dresses a certain way do you think it means that they want your sexual attention or approval?
32. Do you understand that there are many other reasons, that have nothing to do with you, that a person might want to dress or act in a way that you might find sex?
33. Do you think it's your responsibility or role to overcome another person's hesitancy by pressuring them or making light of it?
34. Have you ever tried asking someone what they're feeling? If so, did you listen to them and respect them?
35. Do you think sex is a game?
36. Do you ever try to get yourself into situations that give you an excuse for touching someone you think would say no if you asked? i.e., dancing, getting really drunk around them, falling asleep next to.
37. Do you make people feel "unfun" or "unliberated" if they don't want to try certain sexual things?

38. Do you think there are ways you act that might make someone feel that way even if it's not what you're trying to do?
39. Do you ever try and make bargains? i.e. "If you let me _____, I'll do _____ for you"?
40. Have you used jealousy as a means of control?
41. Have you made your partner(s) stop hanging out with certain friends, or limit their social interactions in general because of jealousy or insecurity?
42. Do you feel like being in a relationship with someone means that they have an obligation to have sex with you?
43. What if they want to abstain from sex for a week? A month? A year?
44. Do you whine or threaten if you're not having the amount of sex or the kind of sex that you want?
45. Do you think it's ok to initiate something sexual with someone who's sleeping?
46. What if the person is your partner?
47. Do you think it's important to talk with them about it when they're awake first?
48. Do you ever look at how you interact with people or how you treat people, positive or negative, and where that comes from/where you learned it?
49. Do you behave differently when you've been drinking?
50. What are positive aspects of drinking for you? What are negative aspects?
51. Have you been sexual with people when you were drunk or when they were drunk? Have you ever felt uncomfortable or embarrassed about it the next day? Has the person you were with ever acted weird to you afterward?
52. Do you seek consent the same way when you are drunk as when you're sober?
53. Do you think is important to talk the next day with the person you've been sexual with if there has been drinking involved? If not, is it because it's uncomfortable or because you think something might have happened that shouldn't have? Or is it because you think that's just the way things go?
54. Do you think people need to take things more lightly?
55. Do you think these questions are repressivve and people who look critically at their sexual histories and their current behavior are uptight and should be more "liberated"?
56. Do you think liberation might be different for different people?

57. How do you react if someone becomes uncomfortable with what you're doing, or if they don't want to do something? Do you get defensive? Do you feel guilty? Does the other person end up having to take care of you and reassure you or are you able to step back and listen and hear them and support them and take responsibility for your actions?
58. Do you tell your side of the story and try and change the way they experienced the situation?
59. Do you do things to show your partner that you're listening and that you're interested in their ideas about consent or their ideas about what you did?
60. Do you ever talk about sex and consent when you're not in bed?
61. Have you ever raped or sexually abused or sexually manipulated someone? Are you able to think about your behavior? Have you made changes? What kinds of changes?
62. Are you uncomfortable with your body or your sexuality?
63. Have you been sexually abused?
64. Has your own uncomfortableness or your own abuse history caused you to act in abusive ways? If so, have you ever been able to talk to anyone about it? Do you think talking about it is or could be helpful?
65. Do you avoid talking about consent or abuse because you aren't ready to or don't want to talk about your own sexual abuse?
66. Do you ever feel obligated to have sex?
67. Do you ever feel obligated to initiate sex?
68. What if days, months or years later, someone tells you they were uncomfortable with what you did? Do you grill them?
69. Do you initiate conversations about safe sex and birth control (if applicable)?
70. Do you think saying something as vague as "I've been tested recently" is enough?
71. Do you take your partners concerns about safe sex and/or birth control seriously?
72. Do you think that if one person wants to have safe sex and the other person doesn't really care, it is the responsibility of the person who has concerns to provide safe sex supplies?
73. Do you think if a person has a body that can get pregnant, and they don't want to, it is up to them to provide birth control? Do you complain or refuse safe sex or the type of birth control you partner wants to use because it reduces your pleasure? Do you try to manipulate your partner about these issues?
74. Are you attracted to people with a certain kind of gender presentation?
75. Have you ever objectified someone's gender presentation?
76. Do you assume that each person who fits a certain perceived gender presentation will interact with you in the same way?
77. Do you find yourself repeating binary gender behaviors, even within queer relationships and friendships? How might you doing this make others feel?
78. Do you view sexuality and gender presentation as part of a whole person, or do you consider those to be exclusively sexual aspects of people?
79. If someone is dressed in drag, do you take it as an invitation to make sexual comments?
80. Do you fetishize people because of their gender presentation?
81. Do you think only men abuse?
82. Do you think that in a relationship between people of the same gender, only the one who is more "manly" abuses?
83. Do you think there is ongoing work that we can do to end sexual violence in our communities?

letter

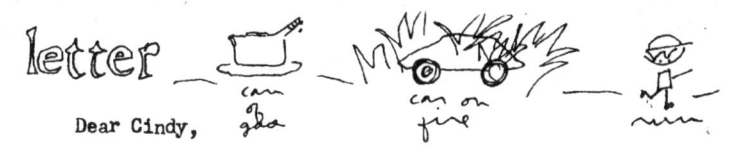

Dear Cindy,

I got your address from Doris #21, which I very much enjoyed reading despite the disturbing subject matter. I myself have never to my knowledge been abused sexually, but somehow its turned out that most of the women I've ever seriously been involved with have. I do not pretend to know how it must feel or what it must do to you mentally, or emotionally. I only really understnad how it can make some people act and react to those close to them. How some things, some emotions are just shut down at times if not closed off all together. And how something as innocent as a kiss can without warning become a nightmare.

The first time I became aware that my girlfriend was abused, I had no idea how to react. I knew her father. Outwardly he seemed like a great guy. I liked him. He let me swim in his pool, and once at a barbeque he gave me a beer (I was only 15) He was aces. Anyway, after we had been seeing eachother for awhile, and things began to become more intimate, she told me about the things he had done to her in the past.

I was stunned. I didn't know how to react, or what to feel. The only real emotion that I could hold on to was anger. I envisioned sneaking up on him late at night with a baseball bat, and beating him stupid. I remember having a whole speech that I would recite while delivering the blows.

Of course I didn't have the nerve to follow through. Instead I set his car on fire. He had a sporty little MR2 that he was very proud of. The ideal midlife crisis mobile. One night he had it parked on the street. I snuck out of my house with a can of gasoline. doused it, and watched it burn from 3 houses away. It looked cool, but ultimately it did nothing to help the situation. It didn't help her, it

didn't help me, and he was heavily insured, so it hardly even buthered him. I realized that no matter how strongly I felt, it just really wasn't my business. Not in that way anyway. Nothing I could do would make it go away.

I never told her what I did. She didn't need revenge. She just wanted me to understand.

Since then I've been involved with several people that have gone through similar ordeals, and although I have never been able to completely empathize with what they went through, I have realized that just listening, and doing all that is possible to maintain a safe, non judgemental, non threatening, and comfortable place where those things can be discussed openly whenever it might come up, is at least a good place to start.

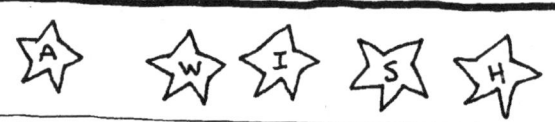

-J

☆A ☆W ☆I ☆S ☆H

"... WHEN HE TOLD ME HE'D BEEN ABUSED AND DIDN'T WANT TO TALK ABOUT IT, I SAID OK. BUT WE WERE BEST FRIENDS FOR FIVE YEARS AND LOVERS FOR ANOTHER FIVE, AND I NEVER BROUGHT IT UP. I REALLY REGRET THAT I DIDN'T ASK HIM ABOUT IT WHEN WE GOT CLOSER."

- S.

"I don't really know how to write about this, but..."

When my partner tells me about her abuse, or things related to it, she becomes really distant and closed off. She talks in a monotone, and it's scary. The stories are hard to hear, and I don't always know what to say or how to reach out to her. For a long time I just didn't know what to do. I would listen. I didn't think I had the right to ask her questions, and I didn't know how to comfort her. I didn't want to make her say more than she wanted to. I didn't want to maker her talk about things she didn't want to talk about.

But I realize that on one hand, she really doesn't want to talk about it all, and on the other hand, she really, really does. She needs to feel like I really want to know, for my own sake, as well as to help her take some of the burden.

Often, after talking about it, she'd be really angry with me. I've learned that even though she needs to talk about it in this distant and removed way, she also needs to let out the feelings, and if I just sit there and listen to her, the feelings of it all still remain bottled up inside.

I'm learning to trust myself more. To try and show her that I care, instead of just acting scared. I ask her if I can hold her, ask what she's feeling, I tell her the monotone is scaring me. Sometimes, this is what she actually needs. She wasn't listened to or believed many times in her life, and sometimes just a few words will bring her back into this time, and she'll see me and recognize that it's me and she'll let me hold her and she'll cry and let out the emotions that go with the story.

But sometimes it's not what she needs. She doesn't want to be held and she gets defensive if I ask what she's feeling. She says things like "What do you think I'm feeling?" She yells.

This used to make me want to run away. It made me feel so worthless, and even now it is hard to understand, but I am starting to see that this anger is part of her healing, part of her protection, and when it happens, I try and not get defensive. I might have to leave, but I try and do it gently - I tell her in a soft voice, a loving voice, that the yelling is scaring me, and that I have to leave for a little bit. I tell her where I'll be and when I'll be back. I don't do it in a threatening way - like I don't tell her to calm down. I just try and accept it all but also, take care of myself.

I always make sure to bring up what happened and to try and learn what's going on, try and show her that I love her and that she's safe, and that I'm willing to do the work, to love her and to know her and to care.

listening

Listening. It's suppose to be this universal thing we all know how to do, but in reality, there are a million different ways to listen. There is listening that is silent, like confession, and listening where you quickly come up with your own opinions, or your own experiences, and like a discussion, you add them in as soon as you get an opening.

Think about listening.
Think about listening. Pay attention to the different ways people you know listen. Figure out what it is that makes you open up to certain people and not others - what qualities of listening do they have? What responses do you need to feel heard?

Of course, everyone is different, and what you need in a listener, most likely won't be the exact same thing that the person you're trying to support will need. But thinking about listening instead of just feeling like it's something we should inherently know how to do, is a first step.

A lot of the times, talking about sexual abuse may need a particular kind of listening. Below are some words about Active Listening, taken from a training manual for rape crisis councilors. (active listening is also used in consensus decision making. It might seem strange and formulaic at first, but it's really a great skill and once you learn to think in this way, it'll stop sounding forced, and will just become part of how you hear and process and listen.

The purpose of active listening is to help you understand what is going on inside the other person. What her feelings are, what she is experiencing, etc. Because that person is not able to always share what's going on inside, the statements she makes are sometimes coded or clouded. This means you have to decode or clear the message, and hear what she is really saying. The only way to know weather you are hearing correctly is to reflect back to the person what you are hearing from her. She will in turn let you know whether you are correct or not.

The purpose is to show that you're interested, that you've not only heard her, but that you understood (or are trying to understand) what she said. It helps check your accuracy of decoding what she's saying. It gives her a chance to breathe. It lets her know that you're actually there. It communicates acceptance. It fosters the person doing their own problem-definition and problem-solving and keeps the responsibility on her, not you.

When an abuse survivor says "I just can't tell anyone what happened", she may be saying any number of things
- I want to forget it ever happened
- I am afraid of what people will think of me
- No one believed me before, why would it be different now
- I am afraid of my feelings about it
- I am afraid I will fall apart if I talk about it
- I am afraid my abuser will come back and hurt me more
- I am afraid you'll think I could have prevented it
- I promised never to tell
- I don't know if I can really trust you

or a million other things

You need to find out the hidden feelings, otherwise you might assume the wrong ones. You can ask "Do you mean..." "Are you saying...", "What does it feel like?"

There are common errors to avoid while active listening, these will bog it down:

exaggerating the feeling, making it more intense than it is. Minimizeing the feeling, not acknowledging it enough. Adding insight into the situation that is not there. Omitting or ignoring things she said to you. Rushing to an insight that the person may be coming to, let her come to it herself. Parroting what she said rather than decoding it. Analyzing what she says, why she feels the way she does.

Characteristics you should have or try to have:

— feeling accepting
— wanting to help
— having and wanting to take enough time
— trusting that she can solve her own problems better than you can

— feeling reasonably separate: (you can empathize with her pain, but don't become disabled yourself.)
— avoid evaluating the person or judging or telling her what to do.
— be aware of your own feelings

DOG DAYZ

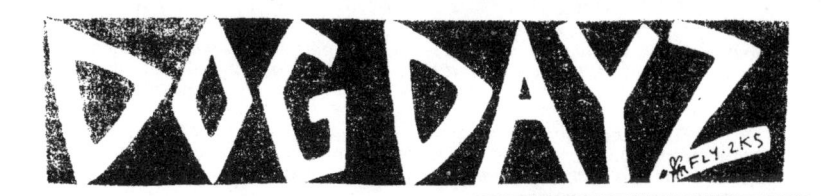

FLY.2K5

"YOU'RE DUMPED!" "WUT!?"
"YOU'RE DUMPED!" "WUT!?"

K9 & DUG HAD STARTED HANGING OUT SOMETIME IN THE SPRING — SHE HAD DUMPED ONE OF HER BOYFRIENDS IN A BAD WAY THAT SHE WAS QUITE ASHAMED OF & THEN — JUST TO BALANCE THINGS OUT — HER OTHER BOYFRIEND HAD DUMPED HER IN A BAD WAY THAT SHE HOPED HE WOULD BE QUITE ASHAMED OF — ANYWAY — SHE HAD HAD ENOUGH OF THOSE SENSITIVE CONCEPTUAL BOYS BECAUSE THEY MADE HER THINK TOO MUCH — THEY MADE EVERYTHING HAVE TO BE EXPLAINABLE & INTENTIONAL WHICH MADE HER NERVOUS — SHE WAS FCKTUP ENOUGH ABOUT SEX WITHOUT HAVING TO ACTUALLY THINK ABOUT IT — WHENEVER K HAD SEX SHE WOULD BE REALLY INTO IT & THEN AT SOME POINT IT WAS LIKE SHE WOULD SUDDENLY BE PARALYZED —

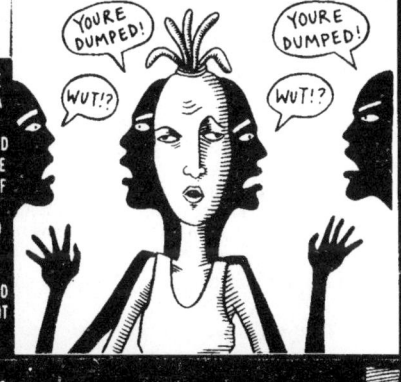

PETRIFIED — USUALLY JUST FOR A FEW SECONDS BUT LONG ENOUGH THAT IT WOULD BE NOTICED BY OTHER INVOLVED PARTIES — SOMETHING HAD HAPPENED A LONG TIME AGO THAT MADE HER WANT TO HAVE SEX BUT ALSO MADE HER AFRAID OF IT & SHE COULDNT REMEMBER ALL THE DETAILS BUT THE IMAGE ALWAYS TOOK OVER AT SOME POINT — SHE WAS BEING SUFFOCATED — SOMETHING BIG & HEAVY ON TOP OF HER — IT WAS HOT & PRICKLY & IT WAS PRESSING HER DOWN SO HARD SHE THOUGHT HER BONES WOULD BREAK & SHE FELT LIKE SHE WAS DYING & BEING BURIED — & THEN SHE WOULD COME BACK & WHOEVER SHE WAS WITH WOULD BE ALL FREAKED OUT & WANTING TO KNOW WHATS WRONG!? WHATS WRONG!? & ALL THAT FCKN CONCERN WOULD JUST MAKE K FEEL LIKE A TOTAL IDIOT — LIKE IF THEY WOULD JUST IGNORE HER THEN MAYBE SHE COULD JUST GET OVER IT BUT THEY MADE HER FEEL LIKE A GODDAM FREAK LIKE SHE HAD TO TALK ABOUT IT & SHE DIDNT WANT TO FCKN TALK ABOUT IT OK!? — CUZ SHE COULDNT FCKN EVEN REALLY REMEMBER IT OK!? -O-FCKN-K!?

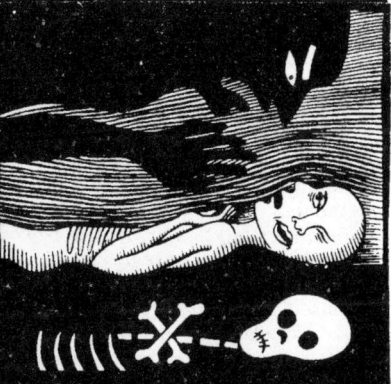

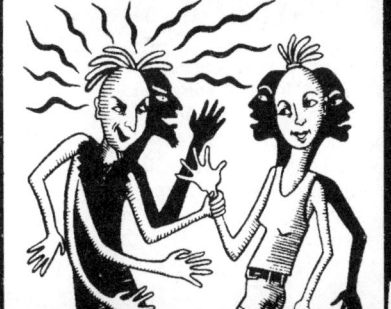

BUT DUG WAS GREAT — HE DIDNT PULL ANY OF THAT ANALYSIS SHIT ON HER — HE JUST GOT INTO THE PHYSICAL STUFF — HE WOULD PLAY FIGHT WITH HER & IT WOULD GET TO A POINT WHERE IT SEEMED SO REAL THAT K DIDNT HAVE TIME TO SPACE OUT — SHE HAD TO STAY AWAKE WITH DUG CUZ HE WAS DANGEROUS & SHE LIKED THAT — K HAD GROWN UP IN A VIOLENT HOUSEHOLD SO LOVE & HATE — SEX & FIGHTING — IT SEEMED LIKE THE RIGHT COMBINATION — & K WAS REALLY HAPPY TO NOT HAVE TO EXPLAIN HERSELF

"Nearly all the survivors I have worked with report having had sex when they didn't want to. It's almost as if this were taken for granted; unwanted sex becomes such a given for survivors that many hardly notice it any more."

"Sometimes there are a number of seemingly contradictory feeling happening in your body at once. You may feel sexually turned on in your hops and vulva, and feel pulled away in your chest.... What do you do then?

Actually, experiencing contradictory feelings is familiar territory for most survivors. Consent then becomes a matter of distinguishing what sensations are what." -The Survivors Guide to Sex (consent and boundaries chapter)

"Survivors are not alone in needing to heal sexually. Our culture leaves little room for people to develop healthy, integrated sexuality. Almost from birth, girls are given mixed messages about their sexuality. They are alternately told to hide it, deny it, repress it, use it, or give it away. The media flaunt sex constantly as a means of power, seduction, and exchange. As a result, most women grow up with conflicts around sex. For women who were abused, these problems are compounded." - Courage to Heal (the chapter in changing patterns: sex)

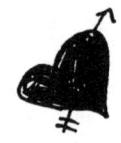

sex etc.

Talking about sex can be really hard - when we were ever taught to talk about it? What language do we use? How do we not feel embarrassed? But really, it is our bodies, it is our lives, it is something that's supposed to be cool and fun and amazing, and why shouldn't we talk about it?

It shouldn't be the responsibility of the person who was abused to initiate conversations about sex.

Spacing out and flashbacks: talking can help. if she looks like she's not present, ask. you could ask her to open her eyes, (don't demand it. just something like "I wish I could see your eyes," or "are you here?") sometimes just a voice can bring us back. sometimes not. it is good to stop or slow down if you are not sure where she is. sometimes you can come up with a code word, like "ghosts" because some people cannot say stop and cannot express what's going on. please don't overreact. don't press her for information. don't feel inadequate. what is appropriate will vary. Sometimes she may want you to leave her alone. sometimes she may want to stay with the flashback and open it up so she can gain information about the past. sometime she will want to be in the present.

You can talk about what, if any, kind of help she might need to stay present. Maybe she needs to say out loud that she wants to be in the present. maybe she needs you to say her name or to tell her who you are or maybe to tell her a story of something simple and nice, not sex related, that you've done together lately. The spiral down can make us forget that there were even nice simple times or any feelings other than fear and helplessness.

When things come up, it can be really important to talk about them again when you're not in bed. You can say "I know you couldn't talk about what was making you so scared and sad last night, but I do really care and really want to know. do you think you can talk about it now?" maybe she'll say yes, maybe she'll say no.

you can say, "It was confusing when I asked if you were ok and you said "I'm fine" but you didn't really sound fine and I didn't know what to do. What should I do when that happens?" maybe she'll say - yeah, she actually was fine, just trying to bring herself back into the present and she was glad you didn't stop and that you trusted her; - maybe she'll say, - yeah, actually, she was saying fine to be cynical, and she's glad you noticed, glad you stopped.

you can say "Do you like it when I _____? I can't tell." maybe she'll say - I want to like it but it makes me feel weird. - maybe she'll say - it's triggering, but I'm trying to work through that trigger. - maybe she'll say - I don't really like that, I just didn't know how to say anything.

If you are courting someone, sleeping with someone, thinking of getting in a relationship with someone, always assume that they could have been sexually abused. Know that for many sexual abuse survivors, even ones who love sex and are aggressively sexual; there will very likely be a period of time when they don't want to have sex. Think about whether you are willing or able to be in a relationship that isn't sexual. It is totally sucky to be an abuse survivor, be emotionally dependent on someone, be having a time of serious abuse triggers, try to set boundaries, try to say you don't want to have sex for awhile, and then have that person freak out or threaten to leave.

If you are willing to be in a relationship that isn't always sexual, (even if you love sex) then it could be a good thing to remind the one you love that if they ever don't want to have sex, it's totally ok.

Every abuse survivor has different needs. They may want to touch you but not be touched. They may want to be touched but not touch you. They may want to have really wild sex. They may want to start over as if they were a teenager and learn to just make out without going all the way. And everything may change at any given moment.

"Your experience of sex can change within a single relationship as well. With a new lover, there's often a passionate rush that obscures problems. But as the relationship settles, sexual issues may need attention again. As you risk more emotional intimacy, you may start to shut down sexually. Or you may find that as your trust grows and deepens, you heal on a deep body level, surpassing even your own expectations.

Because it takes a long time to heal sexually, you may wonder whether you're making progress. But even though the process has ups and downs, you are headed in the right direction. If you are putting steady, consistent effort into developing a fulfilling sexuality, have patience, accept where you are, and trust your capacity to heal." - Courage to Heal

---

terrible. What happen

The first time I ever told the truth about the abuse I experienced, I put all these qualifiers first - saying it wasn't rape or anything, wasn't as bad as what had happened to other people, it was just being touched while I was asleep, and watched while showering and things like that.

The person I was telling it to said "Never compare it. Everyone I've ever met tries to invalidate what happened to them by saying it was worse for someone else. What happened to you was real. What happened to you was terrible. What happened to you counts. Don't belittle it."

This struck me so strongly. I had never believed that I deserved to feel as fucked up as I did about what had happened. That night I practiced writing in my diary, just writing what had happened without any qualifiers, just writing it over and over and finally letting it carry the weight and the pain that it actually did.

SAFE SEX FOR SURVIVORS
by Chris Somerville

Over the past ~~manyzin~~ couple of years I have read as many zines written by sexual abuse survivors as I knew existed. Not a single one had mentioned any comprehensive information or given any tactical ~~INTIM~~ advice about the specific problems that we encounter when we are trying to be sexual. For me, it was my experience of my own sexuality, both in the context of sex with another person and outside of that, which first clued me in to the fact that I had experienced sexual trauma early in my life. After three years of sexual dormancy and thirteen years of repression of memory, I became active again. That's when the flimsy walls of my reality began to really crumble. It was sex that finally released me from the illusion my mind had made in order to keep me safe. It was sex, in a perverted and fucked up form, that inlicted the damage to begin with. And as I moved steadily through a haze of terror, re-entering my sexuality during the onset of my trauma resurfacing, it began to occur to me that sex might end up being at the very core £ of my healing process.

I've known survivors who are too afraid to even think about sex. I've known survivors who have sex constantly and indiscriminantly. We hurt ourselves either way. Sexuality is central to the experience of being human. We NEED to be touched, it's just part of being mammals. The kind of intimacy we are capable of having when we allow ourselves to be open and vulnerable in sex is nourishing down to our very soul. It can reconnect us to our body, rouse emotion we never even knew we could touch, grounds us in present time (what can you think of that brings you into the moment more profoundly than an orgasm?)

I believe that making ourselves vulnerable, truly sharing ourselves, showing our realest selves to another human being is vital for any sucessful healing process.

This is why I believe sex is one of the most effective ways to heal from abuse. You lay naked with someone, with yourself, ~~inxxxxxxxxxxxxxxxxxxxx~~ sometimes you even enter another person's body, take someone inside your own. Isn't that beautiful? It is one of the most powerful experiences a person can have, which is why it can also be so devestating.

I want us to be able to touch this stuff, I don't want to keep avoiding it, living in fear of it becauses of how badly hurt we've been. We still don't know how to do it, though. We can't rely on the culture that raised us to provide any healthy models of sexuality, that's for sure. And we better not wait around for them to address our experiences as survivors either. The best resource we have is eachother. We need to talk to one another, to our friends, our suppor ters, our counselors, our partners, about how to be safe with sex. And we have to not succumb to our fear of sex.

Let's set some terms. First of all, I have no training or expertise of any kind on these matters. All I have to back up what I say here arex my own experiences as a sexually active abuse survivor. When I say "survivor" (which I will, over and over) I am talking about a person who has a sense that she has experienced some kind of sexual trauma at some point in her life. No matter what you remember or what happened, if you feel inside you that this is your experience, you arexx a survivor. Mostly this piece exists for you, it also exists for your partner. When I use the word "partner" I'm not necessarily referring to a serious commited relationship For the purposes if this piece, a partner is anyone you are having sexual contact with on a regular basis. If you're in a place where you're only having one-night-stands, this term still applies.

I am a queer male survivor. The partner who has supported me through the last two and a half years of my recovery is a woman. The gendered nature of the language in this piece is deliberate and is reflected off of my experience. Okay, here we go.

BOTTOM LINES

You don't always get to choose your limits. With my abuse material, I find that I rarely do.
limits tend to set themselves and my task is to work with them, gently pressing up against them whenever I can. We have to be honest with ourselves about what we want, what we can willingly do and what we are unwilling to compromise. These are our bottom lines.

We set our bottom lines based on what we know we need, in sex and in a relationship, without exception.
Naturally, so much of this depends on where you're at with abuse stuff. Here are some examples of what bottom lines might look like:

I cannot get involved with someone who's into SM kmx because I knowx it's retraumatizing for me.

Im only want to sleep with my close friends, I can't be in a serious relationship right now.

My relationship with my partner must be monogamous because it takes so much time and careful attention and trust fer xp me to build a space in a relatioship safe enough in whi ch to be sexual that to allow another person into this space feels like a desecration.

I must have my relationship with my par tner be non-monogamous because any kind of limits imposed on my life or my sexuality by another person reminds me of the entrapment and control I felt during my abuse.

I cannot be in a relationship xixxix with another survivor I can barely hold my own shit together, I can't take on so meone else's.

My partner must be a survivor, too. I don't have the energy or the time to explain myself and explain what I go through to someone who doesn't share my XXXXXXXXXXX experience.

I can't have sex with someone of the same gender as my abuser.

Your bottom lines might not be set up on a scale of polarities the way these ones are, they might not be as "hardline" but it's a really good idea to use words like MUST and CANNOT. Your personal power withhn your own sexuality and your agency within your relationship will both strengthen immeasureably when you decide what you must have, what you can willingly do and what you WILL NOT compromise. Keep in mind that many of these things will change. Some of my bottom lines are the exact oppisite of what they were six months ago. Allow what you need to be malleable but at the same time, understand and respect the fact that what you need right now is what you need RIGHT NOW.

TOUCH YOURSELF

Do not underestimate the far-reaching power of a positive relationship with masturbating. It is a way to explore your ability to have a positive relationship with your body, and it can be a really amazing, strong way to give yourself support with survivor issues.

Masturbating brings our sexual focus back to ourselves,
rather than treating sex as a service to another person.
No one else is there to tell you what they want; your
desires are the only thing on the table. This can be
healing, and can help you to access your right to have
needs.

As sexual child abuse survivors, our first
exposures to sex was entirely on someone else's terms,
following the coercion and fulfilling the needs of our
abuser. Because we learned from the beginning that this

is how sex is supposed to be, we tend
to replicate these patterns now, in our adult sexual
relationships. If we only sexually explore when we're with
another person, we can be strongly influenced by their
desires, or by our own desire to please our partner. We
can confuse this with OUR desires, with what WE
want in sex.

When we shift the focus back to ourselves through masturbating, we retrain our bodies to be sexual for OUR
pleasure and we give ourselves the opportunity to learn
what that means. By fantasizing (aka solo roleplay) and
touching ourselves in different ways, and THEN moving into
the realm of having sex with another person, we build a
source of information and ideas to draw from about what we
want and what's sexy.

Also, and this is really important, if you have rape
fantasies or think about sexually abusing children and are
turned on by this, it's a good idea to fantasize about
these things while masturbating. These feelings need to get
addressed. Masturbating is a great way to do
this because everything you do is on your terms, one hund-
red percent. When these desires aren't aknowledged, are
instead denied and shamed, they begin to become dangerous.
If masturbating while fantasizing about being raped, raping
someone or sexually abusing children only makes you want it
more, it's appropriate to take the next step in bringing it
out into the open by talking to someone and getting some
help.

I believe most survivors need to develop a routine or
ritual by which to get our sexual issues out on the table
and work this material. Masturbating is one of the best
tools we have available to do this because it gives
us the opportunity to heal with our bodies and our minds
simultaneously.

SEX AND POWER

So you've decided to have sex with someone. Congradulations! You're very brave. Now the trick is to figure out a way to have sex in a way that isn't destructive to you or your partner.

The first decision to make is whether or not to tell your ~~partnerxxx~~ partner you're a survivor. You might not feel ~~xx~~ safe enough right away, you might not want him to know at all. Whatever you choose to say, however much you decide to reveal, you should be able to test the waters a little first by dropping a few hints.

For example, explain that you don't want to do certain things in sex because they are TRIGGERING or that you need to establish certain BOUNDARIES in the sex you have together. If he's keen on such survivor lingo as this he'll probably ask more questions and from there you can decide how safe you are to talk about this stuff. If you don't feel safe enough to talk about it then you probably shouldn't have sex with this person.

You need to hold onto your power and establishing your boundaries with a new partner either before you have sex or very early in the sexual phase of your relationship is essential to this. Otherwise you can fall into some pretty nasty sexual power ~~dynamicsxx~~ and feel unable to talk about them.

One particularly hard power dynamic is that of simply not feeling able to have sex. There will likely be times when you don't want to have sex and your partner does, or maybe you want sex in your mind but your body won't allow it. This can be really frustrating for everyone but it's vital that you listen to these messages and accept them. If you attempt to override them, either due to pressure from your partner or from yourself, you can inflict some serious damage. SEX CAN'T BE JUST SEX FOR US. If you are an abuse survivor your relationship to sex CANNOT be the same as that of someone who isn't a survivor.

And to the partners of survivors, as I have been one, I have this to say: If you want to have sex and your partner isn't feeling it, no matter how sudden this may seem, let it end there. Try not to feel rejected because this isn't about you; don't go into your self-hatred,

don't sulk. Wasn't the whole point to feel closer
to this person? Ask yourself what would have happened if
you'd had sex anyway. Is all that hurt and distance and
retraumatization really worth it to have an orgasm?
This should be obvious.

TRIGGERS

A trigger response is when some kind of event or stimulus
causes a person to respond in a way that either regresses
him back to a time in which he was being abused or causes
him to have a sudden, very intense emotional response to
the situation he's in or the person or people he's with.
When you're triggered, your partner can remind you of your
abuser, may even physically resemble your abuser, and you
find yourself removed from present time, experiencing a
flashback of the abuse. Your partner may touch you in a way
that bears no cognitive resemblance to your abuse but may
may suddenly cause you to feel very frightened,
anxious, angry, upset, nauseous, feverish, chilled, or just
very shaken and uneasy.

If you're a survivor and you're sexually active, being
triggered is inevitable, it's going to happen no matter
what. This is okay, triggers aren't bad. They land us in a
temporal state of being afraid and in pain but they happen
when it's time for us to confront an aspect of our abuse.
A trigger is a message from our system letting us know what
we need to be paying attention to and working on right now.

But triggers are still scary and really intense, so it's
important that each of us devise a response system to being
triggered so we can have a clearer idea of what to do when
it happens. This is something we can do alone and with our
partners. I would recommend doing both.

A good thing to do after you've calmed down from the
initial flurry of being triggered, but with the experience
still fresh in your mind and body, is to write a list of
questions you ask yourself in order to figure out what you
need when this happens. For example: Am I disassociating
right now? (more on this later) Do I need to come back
into my body? Do I need to be with my partner? Do I need to
be held? Do I need to not be touched? Do I need to be
alone? Is there someone else I want to talk to right now?
Do I need to just lay still? Do I need some water? Do I
need to eat something? Do I need to get up and move around? Do I need to meditate? Do I need a cigarette?

Laminate your list of questions with packing tape and keep it close to the place you have sex, under your pillow, in the drawer where you keep your sex toys and condoms, wherever you can get to it when you need it. Make sure your partner knows where it is or has a copy himself.

So you've been triggered. The first thing to do is to notice the feeling you're having and if you can, name it. "I feel afraid," "I feel dirty and gross," "My stomach hurts really bad," "I'm going to cry," You may feel an urge to ignore what's going on inside you and just keep going. FIGHT THIS! Say that you need to stop. Now your partner asks, "what do you need?" If he doesn't ask you this, tell him anyway. You might not know exactly what you need. Look for that great list you made and try to find out this way, ask yourself all the questions on the list. If you're still not sure what you need or if you don't have a list, just try to be still and stay present with your feelings. This may be all that you need right now.

To the person supporting the triggered survivor: The focus needs to be on your partner in this situation. He needs to be the one calling the shots because he's the one having the discomfort. As survivors are people who have had their power taken away over and over again, a supportive partner needs to do just that: support him. Don't try to fix or rescue him, he needs to take that power back for himself, to make the situation better for himself. Stay present with him, hold the space in tact.

DISASSOCIATION

When a survivor disassociates she may not be having any intense feelings like would be found in a triggered response, she is simply gone, not in her body, not present in her experience. This response is less alarming than a trigger response but it is just as serious. There is still a way to return to present time.

It's hard to disassociate when you're looking into someone's eyes. This can be awkward and scary and hard; it can also be incredibly intimate and can do a lot to keep you present in your body. The partner of a survivor is more likely to notice his partner disassociating than the survivor will notice herself.
Ask "are you here?" or "where are you?" And be very gentle with this. Make it safe for her to come back.

These are only the simplest of tools, only a skeleton of a support system. The real substance of any functional ~~XXXXXXXXXXXXX~~ method of healing is .. based on a dedication to caring for yourself and a strong bond with those you love. So take care of eachother, and be patient. This stuff takes a long time. As a survivor, I know that my experience of myself, of my relationships and of my sexuality is profoundly different from the experience of someone who was not sexually abused. And this is okay. It's okay for us to have to work hard at what other people take for granted. The goal is not to return to some arbitrary centerpoint of normalcy from which we were robbed as children. We are not deviants. The goal is to heal, to be on a continuum of healing. I am not asking for what I had before, I am asking only for redemption.

Write to me!
Chris Somerville
509 Garrison St. NE
Olympia, WA 98506

And special thanks to Laura for all the good ideas.

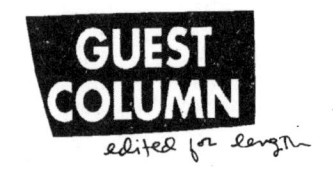

GUEST COLUMN *edited for length*

By Anandi *reprinted from MRR*

... I want to talk about what I see coming up in our lives so often, which are casual encounters. Like for example, maybe you guys are drunk and you start making out at a party. Or you've been flirting for a while, and go on a date and finally start making out. What I mean is, you don't really know each other super well yet, and it's just not time for the big talk, you know? Like, maybe after, or next time, you'll start talking and tell each other things about your histories or whatever, but by then it might be too late; you might've already totally freaked this person out by maybe unknowingly acting like a total dick.

Some stuff should be obvious. If someone says, "I don't want to be sexual" and then you put your hand in their pants while they're asleep, well... you're a creep, and you're not even trying to *not* be one. But! I think even the biggest creeps can change! ... I'm going to assume that the majority of people reading this are good people, and that if you're making out with someone, it's to be fun for both of you, you want them to be happy, you don't want to cause them pain. So I'm going to try to help you, so no one need ever say again, "I didn't know! How could I have?

...If you think you have never been with someone with a history of abuse or rape, it is much more likely that you simply aren't coming across as someone who people feel they can tell these things to. You might read this and think, well, that's not my friend, I know they can take care of themselves! Like as if some girl who throws bottles at cops (or whatever) would definitely be able to say no! But that is not so! ... Actually a person can be very outspoken and still be unable to stick up for themselves sexually. And in fact, survivors of violence are very often these very same tough-as-hell seeming people.

...Aside from the practical advice part of this, the how to make out with someone without unknowingly causing them to relive their histories of abuse or just be a jerk, I want to say a few things. One is that, no matter what you think about all this, whether you think you need this advice or not - consider this! If you take my advice and you treat everyone in this way, you will be so popular! People will tell each other, oh, s/he was so sweet and great and...do you see where I'm going with this? I'm trying to say you'll be better in bed, OK?? And everyone will want to get it on with you!

Another is that just because you're a girl doesn't mean you can't do things to people that might be triggering or putting pressure on them... Same goes for survivors of abuse. Being a victim does not make it impossible for you to victimize, and in fact we are statistically much more likely to pass on our fucked up shit... And! just because you do it only with boys doesn't mean you don't need to worry about these thing either. Yes, more girls that guys are sexually victimized in this society, but given that pretty much every girl I know has some kind of fucked up story, that's not saying much. And the fact is, it can be even harder for male victims to talk about these things, that there may be even less space where they can feel safe dealing with these issues, and even less consideration for their pain. So please, be careful with everyone, OK?

The absolute, number one most important thing is to pay attention to the person you're with! Even if you're really drunk, or really turned on, or both. If you can't tell if they're into it or not, if they're being real quiet, Stop! It is your job to stop if you suspect your partner is not having fun! The most sure sign you will ever get that something is definitely wrong is if the person who you're with seems to change suddenly, to become quiet or more withdrawn, tenses up, stops looking at you, or anything that makes you feel more alone suddenly. Do Not assume they are all right! And then, don't just hear what you wanna hear. If you stop and then you say "hey, you OK?" well sure, pat yourself on the back for being so rad if you need to, but then! If the person you're with kinda looks down or up or off to the side and says real quiet like, "no it's nothing don't worry, I'll be fine," you know something? It is not OK to be like, "well, I tried, no one can say I didn't, so fuck it." I mean, do you like this person or not?! Sex is supposed to be fun! For both of you! You can tell the difference between someone who's having fun and someone who isn't, I know you can. The problem is that most people second guess themselves, they think, well, I must be wrong, it must just be how this person is, maybe she's always quiet, or it must be fine because he's a dude and guys always want to have sex, and because otherwise they'd say something, right? Well, no. Not necessarily.

One of the first and most common causes of misunderstandings in a sexual context, and one of the most pervasive side effects of any kind of abuse history, is many survivors' inability to stick up for themselves in the ways that matter most. Abuse, especially if it happened when we were children (...or teens) teaches us that it doesn't matter what we want, it won't be respected, and if we don't say anything we don't have to face the fact that that is what is happening. If we say no, and someone does what they want to our body anyway, we have to fact the fact that a violation has occurred. However, if we don't say anything we can later say to ourselves, "well, they didn't know, so they aren't so bad and I don't have to deal with the things I would have to if I admitted to myself what I know and feel, which is that they should have known, and that I secretly hate them." ... The person you're making out with may be actually literally unable to advocate for themselves, to say to you, please stop. Please don't. They may be frozen by the fear that you will not like them anymore, or that you may think that they don't like you, or they may just be so far inside themselves that they cannot do anything.

Because that is what happens. We freeze. Basically what happens to most of us when something is going on that reminds us of the bad things that have happened to us in the past is that we shut down, mentally and emotionally. We turn inward so that we do not have to experience the things that are happening to our bodies, because it is so painful emotionally and/or physically, and so terrible, to have someone disregard you in this way. It's kind of hard to explain, but anyone who has been through this sort of thing can tell you that it's true. And your goal is not to cause anyone to have to do this, every, because it is a terrible, traumatizing feeling. If you do this to someone, it's fucked up, even if it was not on purpose....

Which brings up the other really big thing. If someone tells you something about their personal experiences with sexual trauma, however unlikely it may seem, you must believe them. Period. If someone says to you, "if you touch my elbow while I'm kissing you I will freak out," I don't care how silly it seems to you, just don't do it! And furthermore, try really hard to understand, to really understand that it's important. ... and it won't always be as easy as that, their needs might cost you something. Like this person you're hooking up with might say "I can't have intercourse, and also I can't go down on you." And you might think, "but that's the only way I can come," but you are gonna have to figure something out, because it's really really not OK for you to try to talk them into it, even by telling them how gentle and how great you'll be about it. You must respect them and their needs! It is not easy for a survivor (or just a girl in general in this society) to reach the point where they can even figure out what it is that they need, let alone tell you, so for god's sake, take it seriously when they can!

It's not easy to do these things. Mostly, it's really hard to learn how to be truly present in sexual situations. But it is possible, and I think it's desirable to try to change the way we are with relation to sex... This is something our society just doesn't teach us how to do or encourage us to learn, and in a way we are all survivors of the fucked up things we're taught about sex. We learn that we're suppose to want it all the time, but also that it is shameful. We are bombarded with sexual imagery every day, yet we are told that we shouldn't talk about sex, especially not honestly; that sex is only okay to talk about if it's in alienating gross ways that aren't good for anyone's sexuality. And so lots of times we're so busy trying to prove something that we can't just relax and have fun, and ... I think everyone can benefit from thinking about this stuff.

And while it doesn't come naturally, neither does relating to each other in these fucked up ways. We were able to learn that; we can unlearn it. It isn't something that happens all at once; it is a constant process, even for someone who thinks about this stuff all the time. But it can happen!

A couple other random things --

---It's great to ask people what's up and be ready to talk to them about it, but if they're not ready or up to talking about it, please respect that too. It doesn't help to be all macho about your new role as a supportive partner and go around demanding that people open up and share with you, right now!

---Try not to take in personally if your partner says, "yes, actually I am feeling freaked out and I don't want to do this right now." Don't give the person a guilt trip. They're having a hard time already and probably a lot of guilt issues too.

---One thing doesn't not mean or imply another. If someone says the are OK with kissing, it doesn't mean they are OK with being felt up, etc. It means they are OK with kissing.

---Just use protection. Your partner shouldn't have to ask, and they damn sure shouldn't have to argue about it. And if you can't get it together enough to carry any....then accept that you may not get to do certain things as a result. No arguing!

---OK, this is a tricky one, and you all can write me and tell me how fucked up I am...but listen -- If you're under 30 and you're dating someone who is more than five years younger than you, then consider the possibility that there may be a serious power imbalance in your relationship, which probably rules out any possibility of honest communication. You may think you're different, and you may really be, but everyone thinks their relationship is the 1% that is fucked up, and 99% of them are wrong, you know? I spent my whole teenage years dating people much older than me, and ... saying that it wasn't like that, but it wasn't until I had a boyfriend of my own age for the first time when I was 19 that I realized how different it was to be in an actual relationship of equals where I felt like I could actually speak. Does my experience men everyone is like this? No, of course not, but I've talked to plenty of other punk girls who know exactly what I'm talking about and have the same history. And an unequal dynamic means that the chances of someone enduring sex that they are not comfortable with or that may be damaging to them are increased many many time over.

She had slept with a lot of people. It made me feel inadequate as a lover. I wish I'd been more sure of myself, because I think I made her feel like I judged her just like everyone else did, like I thought she was a slut, when she was only trying to survive and figure things out.

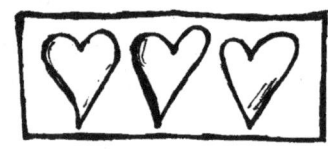

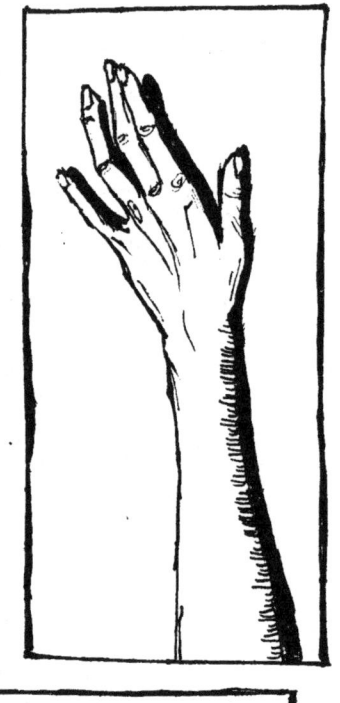

ME AND ALISON HAVE BEEN TOGETHER 15 YEARS. EVERY ONCE AND AWHILE WE'LL ARGUE AND IT MAKES HER REALLY DOOMED, SAYING THINGS LIKE "THIS IS ALWAYS WHAT HAPPENS! IT'S NOT WORTH IT! WHY DON'T YOU JUST LEAVE!" WE LOVE EACH OTHER SO MUCH, BUT ITS HARD TO HOLD ON TO MY SELF CONFIDENCE WHEN SHE SAYS THINGS LIKE THIS. I TRY TO STEP BACK AND NOT LET MYSELF GET TOO WRAPPED UP IN THOSE EMOTIONS AND I TRY TO LOOK LOGICALLY AT IT AND REALIZE THAT SHE'S SO HURT, AND I TRY AND EXPLAIN WHY OUR RELATIONSHIP IS DIFFERENT FROM OTHER ONES, AND HOW WE CAN MAKE IT THROUGH ALL THIS.

I helped him write letters to his family, and answered the phone so he wouldn't have to talk to them until he was ready.

I hate it when people say "whenever you want to talk about it, I'll be there." I fucking never want to talk about it. I hate it. But I need to talk about it. I need them to want to hear. I need them to actually make an effort to bring it up, even if it's scary. I don't understand why they're not more curious. I would be. I would want to know. I swear to god, it's scarier for me then them.

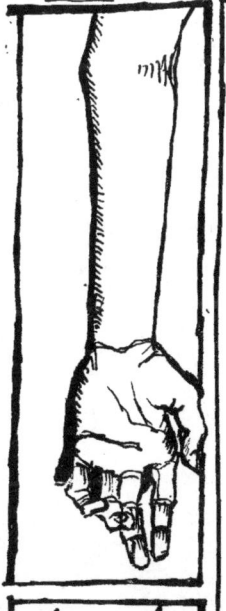

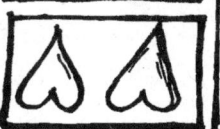

Whenever he would get sad and overwhelmed by abuse memories, it would make me sad too, and then he'd have to be the one to get us both out of it by changing the subject or ending something. He told me that—it made him feel like he should never show his feelings, because he didn't want to make me feel bad. So now even when I feel sad because of him feeling sad, I try to make an effort to not let it consume me, and to try and focus on what he's feeling and needing. I can always feel the sad stuff some other time.

It feels weird to repeat myself over and over, but that's what she need and so that's what I do. I feel sort of self-conscious, but I just tell her over and over that it wasn't her fault and that she's good. I mean it. She really is the most amazing person I've ever known.

When I start to apologize for being fucked up, that's when I need more comfort but can't figure out how to get it. If I'm apologizing a lot, then I know I need to get out of that relationship or situation.

different needs

I was sexually abused when I was a young girl, and so was pretty much ever girl I've dated. And all of us have needed really different things. I used to be really "strong" and didn't like to talk about it at all, and when people used to push me to talk about it, it was actually just really bad for me, but now I like it when people ask me if it's ok before they touch me in certain ways, or just to check in when we're making out, but my current girlfriend hates the word "ok". I mean, she doesn't mind asking me, but for her, "is this ok?" makes her feel defensive and like - of course, everything's fine. She can survive anything. I guess sort of like when parents are worried about you, and they ask if you're ok when you're just really obviously not. So those words make her leave her body, but if I say "Do you want this", that works for her.

Another girlfriend really didn't want to be asked any questions. She just really needed me to pay close attention and to be able to notice if she was fazing out, and then to just stop and hold her.

A lot of the girls I've been with really don't want to or can't be monogamous. This is hard for me, because I really do like just being the only one, and I have jealousy problems that I'm struggling with, and I guess some of my stuff relates back to the abuse and how things were done to my body, and my body wasn't loved or treasured or protected; and I just feel so bad about my body and about myself most of the time, I just want someone to commit to only me, and to love me so much they don't want anyone else. But I also understand where they're coming from. I understand how monogamy can feel like someone owning and controlling your body, and I totally understand needing to not feel owned.

For a long time, I've struggled to be ok with non monogamy, but I think from now on, I should probably talk about it before getting into a relationship, and that I should possibly take it in to consideration, and maybe not go out with girls who don't want to be monogamous, because it always ends up just being such a painful and hard struggle, when we already have so much to contend with. It's hard though, because when I like someone, and am in that amazing, crushed out, beginning time, the last thing I want to do is talk about this kind of thing.

I think one of the other really extremely hardest things I've had to figure out how to deal with, is when I think everything is going fine, and then my girlfriend will tell me that actually something was really wrong. Like she didn't actually want to have sex the last few times that we did. Or that she was faking orgasms. Or that something I do is triggering.

This is just the worst feeling, and it is so hard not to just panic and be like - "why didn't you tell me!" I really did say that once, in this sort of accusatory voice, "You never told me!" It feels so terrible to have done this. I am trying to be really good, and I know it is just that she is so used to pretending, because that's just been her defense mechanism for years, but it is still horrifying that I have added to unwanted shit in her life.

So when this happens, it is really hard not to get scared and sort of not on purpose, blame her for letting it happen. But really, I know that this is the worst thing I could do, and I am trying to figure out how to feel just happy that she's finally telling me, and that she feels safe enough to tell me, and then maybe I can comfort her and when it's appropriate we can figure out ways to try and not let it happen again. But even if we figure out ways, sometimes they don't work, and we just have to keep talking, and caring, and supporting each other.

Dear Cindy,

I wanted to write and thank you for Doris #21 - it is kick-ass and brave and one of the only things that has really woken me up in a long time. I also wanted to give you my thoughts, reactions and story before I lost my nerve and in case any of it is useful for your zine.

I haven't thought about any of this stuff consciously in a long while, have spent the last 5 years trying to stuff it under the surface. After 10 years of therapy, I can only say that "something bad" happened with an older male family member. In my 20's I tried to pull at those threads and

unravel them, and I had terrible panic attacks and depression on and off for years. My family disowned me and I caved. Now I am living a split life, in contact with my family and pretending nothing happened while knowing inside that it did. After that early experience, I got into many other bad situations with men because I was so numbed out and unaware that I could want anything.

What's always hurt me is that I wanted to do political organizing around womens issues and never could. It's mysterious, but being with a group of women always triggers because something about rape or assault will come up and I'll feel for a few days like I'm drowning and I can't breath. I have responded to the whole sexual assault thing by being very tough and no-nonsense in my activist and job lives, and being with women makes me feel things, makes me feel vulnerable and then I feel crazy because I lose control. It's weird, I have wanted more than anything to be politically active with a group of women, but because I want it so much, I get intimidated when I get near real women I admire. If I don't have a sense that they've gone through something similar, I get afraid they will reject me for being damaged, and if they <u>have</u> been through something similar, I get afraid they'll talk about it too much and I'll get triggered. I don't know, my relationships with women are fulfilling but complicated, I think partially because my mom "sold me out" on numerous occasions and chose the abuser over me.

Being assaulted has taken a lot from me. I get triggered all the time and have 1000 tricks that no one knows for keeping it together. Even at activist conferences, there are

creepy men and I find myself panicking and being defensive and silent instead of speaking up and telling them to get the fuck away. I had EMDR treatment a few years ago, which really helped and has taken some of the edge off of my startle reflex.

I loved your zine because you reminded me that this is political. I always forget that, or I know it for other people but not for me.

Having been assaulted means I have a fucked-up relationship to activism sometimes. I take on too much and say yes to too much because I think I'm not worthy or even alive unless I'm in pain and panicked and doing too much for other people.

Being an assault survivor in a movement of anarcho-socialists and socialists is a weird thing. For example, people gave me weird looks when I got married and took my partner's last name, like "ooh, you sellout." Screw that - I could explain to almost no one that I was overjoyed to get rid of the last name that linked me to my abuser. I just went from one man's name to another, and at least I love my husband. I think even in movements that call themselves radical, there are a lot of judgements about women and a total lack of understanding a about what real women have to do to make it through the day.

This has also gotten really bizarre and important since I found out I'm going to be the mom of a boy. I tried to admit to some movement people that that was a weird thing for

me, but they looked at me like I was being vicious. I think for any feminist, the challange of raising a good man is daunting and mysterious. For a sexual assault survivor, it is... well, for me at least it's alternately hopeful and very scary. It's a huge and beautiful challange that might give me the first experience of loving a male completele and safely and unconditionally. But I doubt my own abilities and I don't

want to look at my son ever when I'm triggered or down on men and make him feel like I hate him just because he has a penis. But I will NOT raise him to be one of those smug shitters who is so "I'm a feminist" that he never listens and can never be wrong. I've seen more of those, including "radical" ones, than I've met decent radical men. One of the reasons I'm really into my husband is because he's a normal working class guy who knows men can be fucked up, not a holier-than-thou radical who wants to lecture me on being more "strong" or "feminist".

I feel like I've been working so hard for years to rise above this stuff and build a life and stay alive. And that's

my weird secret, because I tell almost no one these days. But it is so important to talk about and acknowledge and to give myself credit for dealing with it. Hopefully someday there will be a way to express this stuff out in the open. Thank you for letting in some air.

"I never thought I'd feel safe enough to just lay around all sleepy at a big old party like this."

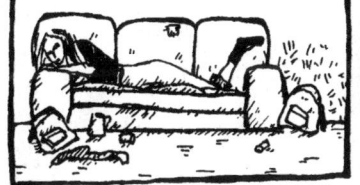

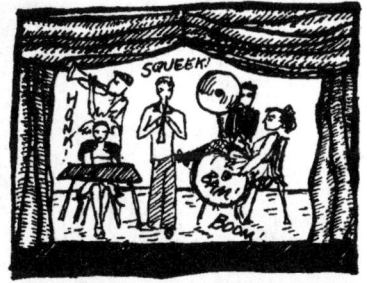

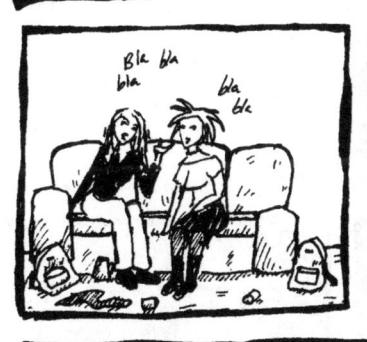

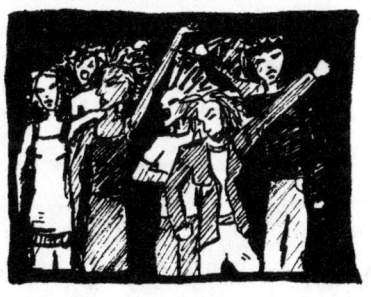

Bla bla bla / bla bla

I didn't always feel so safe...

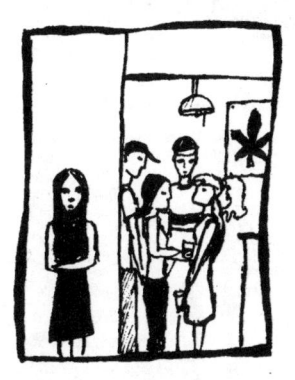

I grew up in a college town. There was a football stadium down the street that looked like a castle.

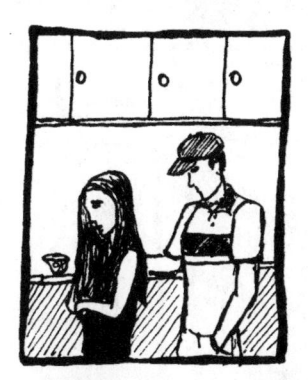

We were kids and we would go to parties. There was always something about these parties that made me uneasy...

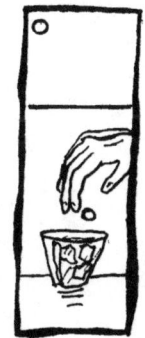

...like I was surrounded by predators.

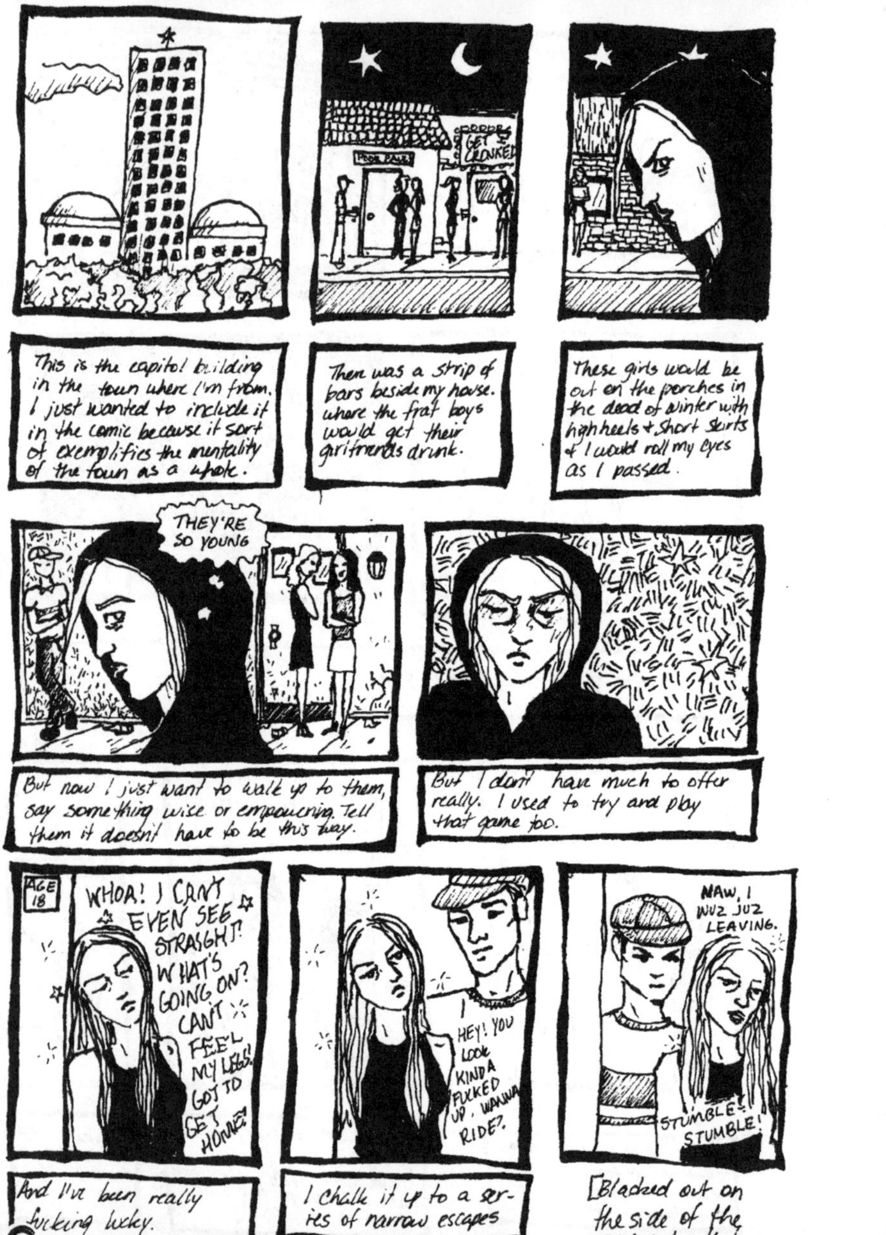
This is the capitol building in the town where I'm from. I just wanted to include it in the comic because it sort of exemplifies the mentality of the town as a whole.
There was a strip of bars beside my house. where the frat boys would get their girlfriends drunk.
These girls would be out on the porches in the dead of winter with high heels + short skirts + I would roll my eyes as I passed.
THEY'RE SO YOUNG
But now I just want to walk up to them, say something wise or empowering. Tell them it doesn't have to be this way.
But I don't have much to offer really. I used to try and play that game too.
AGE 18
WHOA! I CAN'T EVEN SEE STRAIGHT! WHAT'S GOING ON? CAN'T FEEL MY LEGS! GOT TO GET HOME!
And I've been really fucking lucky.
HEY! YOU LOOK KINDA FUCKED UP. WANNA RIDE?
I chalk it up to a series of narrow escapes
NAW, I WUZ JUZ LEAVING.
STUMBLE! STUMBLE!
[Blacked out on the side of the road. later that evening]

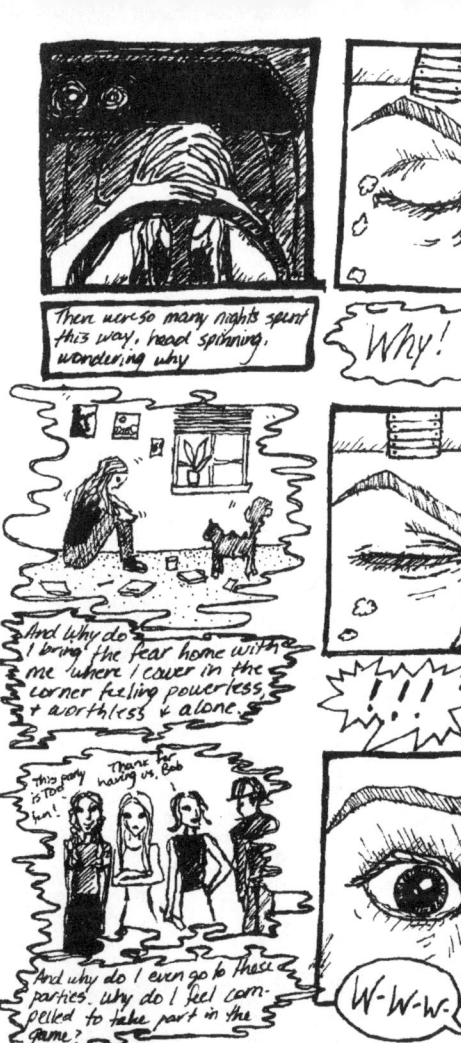

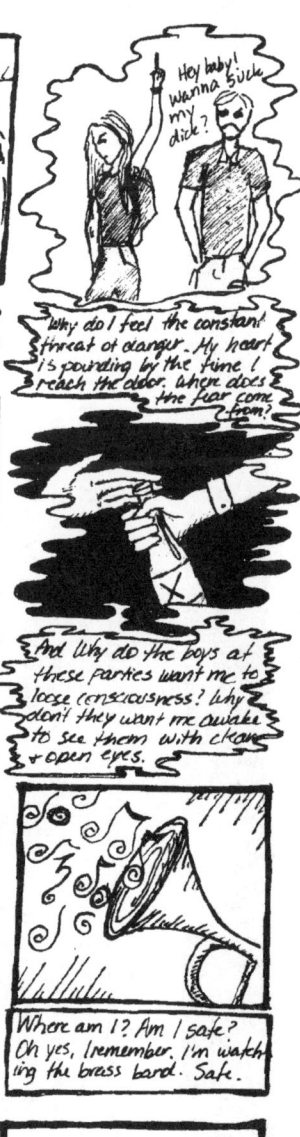

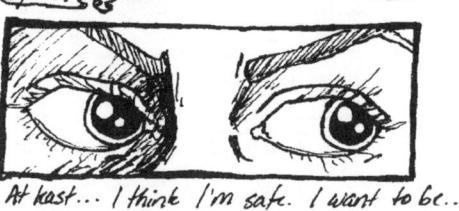

Then were so many nights spent this way, head spinning, wondering why

Why!

"Hey baby! Wanna suck my dick?"

Why do I feel the constant threat of danger. My heart is pounding by the time I reach the door. Where does the fear come from?

And why do I bring the fear home with me where I cower in the corner feeling powerless, & worthless & alone.

!!!

And why do the boys at these parties want me to loose consciousness? Why don't they want me awake to see them with clear + open eyes.

"This party is Too fun!" "Thanks for having us, Bob"

And why do I even go to these parties. Why do I feel compelled to take part in the game?

W-W-W-

Where am I? Am I safe? Oh yes, I remember. I'm watching the brass band. Safe.

At least... I think I'm safe. I want to be...

Fin

by Janet

I grew up constantly reminded of abuse. My mother was a public health nurse who frequently examined children for signs of abuse or neglect. She never censored her work stories from me even when I was very young. I remember being about 5 years old when my mother told a particularly gruesome story at dinner one night. My sister, 9 years older, got up and said, "I don't want to hear about this stuff," and left. I stayed, big-eyed, listening to my mother tell tales of cigarette burns, beatings, and molestation.

Do I think she shouldn't have told me those stories? Not necessarily. But I do remember feeling more than upset for the children she spoke of; I felt guilty. Maybe it was my Southern Baptist upbringing, but I felt guilty that my own childhood was so relatively peaceful and free from violence. Why did these other kids have so much worse things to deal with? Why didn't I?

Remembering that guilt is important for me when I deal with friends who have been sexually abused. Their stories weigh on me. So many abused by brothers, step brothers and cousins, one raped by her grandfather, one molested by her mother, one the resident sex toy for family and friends—the list goes on and on. But that didn't happen to me. I may have had my share of abusive encounters since childhood but I wasn't abused as a child. I was never raped by a stranger or by someone I was in a relationship with.

Often when I hear my friend's stories or I read about a woman stalked, raped or killed in the paper, I think, "Why them? Why not me?" There's a name for that feeling; psychologists call it survivor guilt. It's the horrible feeling the people who survive a terrible event are left with. It was first identified after the Holocaust when many people who escaped the camps expressed severe guilt for having survived the camps when their friends and family members had not. This guilt and the horrors they'd seen led many survivors of the camps to kill themselves years after their escape. People who survive accidents, disasters, and combat when friends or family have died are also prone to survivor guilt.

Given these scenarios, it makes sense to me that in our society, many women would feel this extreme guilt. We live in state of constant surveillance from the male gaze. We have to think about our safety whenever we make choices about where we go or how we get there. We are inundated with tales of assault, abuse, and the murder of women. Of course those of us who survive to see another day would feel guilt. Constantly confronted with tales of sexual violence, one would feel not only fear but also a sense of "that could've been me" and maybe even "why wasn't that me?" What I want to look at here is how those feelings manifest themselves when I deal with abuse. What does acute awareness of abuse do to me and how does it affect how I treat people who are working through abuse issues?

I. Support is a tricky business

When I first find out a friend has been abused, I sometimes grow apprehensive, I get a sort of "walking on eggshells" feeling. I want so badly to be supportive, to say or do the right things. This reaction has positive and negative aspects. It's good to be careful with your friends, especially when they are having a hard time. But treating your friend like she is a very fragile creature can be alienating because that's not the whole story. Many people who have been abused may be fragile in some ways but they are also very strong in other ways. Treating them as if they may fall apart at any instance means not acknowledging their resilience. They've been through so much, yet they are still going. Recognizing the strength it takes to confront abuse, not just sympathizing with the stories, is a vital part of supporting someone who has been abused. Sometimes the pain of hearing the story of someone you love makes this easier said than done, but it's important.

II. The trickier part

Sometimes support doesn't mean just listening and nodding in sympathy. Sometimes being a friend means challenging your friends even if you think the behavior in question may stem from abuse. Women in our culture can easily grow up thinking that their only worth is that of an object of sexual desire. Imagine how much that belief would be amplified if you were sexually abused as you developed your idea of who you are and what you are here for.

After my own rocky adolescence, I came away from a series of lame sexual encounters with a defiant "use or be used" attitude towards sex. If sex was all I was worth, then I would use it to my advantage. Years later, a healthy sexual relationship showed me what a negative framework I had been using—one rife with fucked up power dynamics. I'd like to think that acknowledging my own power issues with sex would lead to me discussing them with friends who also seem to be dealing with the same issues. And sometimes I do. But, I've found that if my friend has been sexually abused, I'm less likely to bring them up. If I see sexual manipulation, an extreme need for male attention, competitiveness with women, or any other behavior I might be able to link to their abuse history, chances are I won't say anything. My general thought being, "they're dealing with enough already." This

First of all, if the behavior that bothers me is actually connected to my friend's abuse history, she may want to think about that connection. Healing happens when you can look at all parts of your life, how you treat people, how you see yourself. Not talking to someone about their behavior denies them an outside perspective and a chance to work on some of their issues. I'm not doing them a favor by ignoring the possible effects of abuse.

More importantly, maybe I'm wrong. Women from all types of backgrounds exhibit the behaviors I mentioned earlier, we're brought up that way. What if my friend's actions don't stem from abuse. Maybe if I talk to them I'll see that there is no connection. I'll see I've committed that grave error psychologists often commit, tracing everything back to a starting place, a seed in childhood. Not talking to her keeps me from straightening out my own skewed perceptions. Maybe I'm attributing too much to a part of my friend's life. Maybe their actions come from a million other motivations and forces that have nothing to do with abuse. A person is much more that the bad things that have happened to them. To assume that all their actions stem from past traumatic events is reductive and unfair. By not talking about abuse and its possible effects, I deny my friend the chance to tell me how she perceives her self and her world. This lack of communication reinforces the silencing effects of abuse. Support means talking more, even when it's difficult. I suppose it seems facile to say "we all need to talk more," but we do. Let's bring stuff up, abuse related and otherwise. Let's challenge each other, listen, and learn.

Dear Cindy

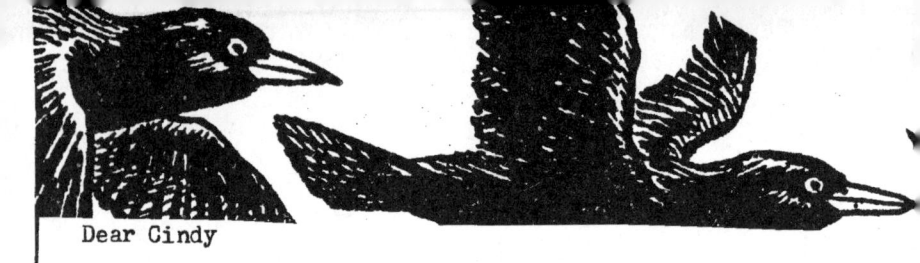

... I read your column for Slug and Lettuce. Oh, I love the way it is angry and questioning, very direct and clear in the anger. yeah, I was at Nove Miasto and asked some of the guys there to read it, and they complained about how small the print was so I went and photocopied it BIG and then they didn't have any excuses. but lets not talk about excuses. I am glad that you wrote such a moving piece, it makes me feel ok when I've been questioning lately how I "let" certain situations happen. but fuck that. I have been so conditioned, trained, and taught my entire life that whatever he says, goes, and that it is more important to be sexy and liked by the guys than building lasting honest relationships with people...

I've been thinking and writing about all these situations/ stories from my life that have reinforced a patriarchy deep deep within my head. and it's really making me split wide open as I start to understand where it's been coming from and how I perpetuate it. It's exciting, kinda; I can see how I am moving away from it and challenging behaviors that wreck me. and maybe, also, I'm just over it. Maybe I'm finally realizing that being boy-crazy ain't where it's at, that random fucking hurts and leaves me bruised, and that no kinda boyfriend/soulmate/partner will complete me and provide my happiness. In some ways it seems like so much work to break out of these patterns, but I'm also feeling a big sense of relief and excitement at letting go. ...

love, sarah

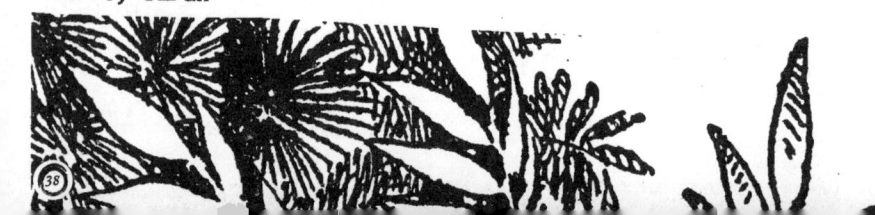

FROZEN INSIDE reprinted from Slug and Lettuce

I can't believe how the fuck it keeps happening; people waking up to someone they know touching them. How the hell can anyone think it is ok to initiate sex with someone who is sleeping?

Do they think about our abuse histories? Or the fact that we can't say "no" when we're asleep? Do they understand our complex defense systems and how vulnerable and terrified we might feel waking up to this assault? Do they know that even if we go along with it all, once we wake up, it doesn't necessarily mean we wanted to? We have complex ways of protecting ourselves. Do they think about this?

The truth is, I used to crawl in people's beds too. I thought it was ok. I thought of course all guys wanted it. I never considered the fact that I might be capable of assault. But of course, I am. A lot of us are.

Are you seeing this? Will you promise to take steps to never do it again?(like don't get in bed with someone when you're wasted or unsure about your intentions. Stop making excuses for yourself. Look at your life for real.)

I am sick of how it all keeps happening. I can't stand how often people tell me something like this: "I told him, early in the night, that just because we were getting drunk together didn't mean I wanted to fuck him. I specifically said 'I don't want to have sex with you" and then later, he was just on me. Do we call this rape?"

Or how many times I've heard "I didn't say no outright, but I tried to make it clear." And then there are all the times we try to comfort someone or find comfort in their arms, and they think it's an invitation to do what they want. We trust people and they don't understand (or care?) about the difference between emotional openness and sexual desire. Or how it happens; if we're slutty or flirty people think we're open game. If we're shy, they think it's a form of flirt and really they just need to be persistent in pressuring us. This game is not always a fun game for all of us.

Yesterday, a tough girl friend of mine said "I have not had consensual sex all year." The day before I heard friends laughing about two people we knew who had been wrestling and one of them had just thought it was comraderie until the other person ...

and everyone is laughing at the story because it is a boy - boy story, which I don't think is funny at all.

The day before that I was reading a zine where she's calling someone out. She says "That was assault, asshole!" but at the end of the page it says "I should have fought."

I am sick of people saying, "well, if you didn't want it, why didn't you say something. I never would have had sex (or whatever(with you if I'd known."

I am sick of the blame and self blame. We have had practically everything taken away from us and can not always speak. And what kind of world are we building? If it's still seen as our responsibility to say something? Why isn't it their responsibility to ask and watch for signs and signals, and ask again?

You know how there are supposedly two instinctual responses -- fight or flight? Well, there's also freeze. you can see it everywhere in nature, especially in animals that are under constant attack.

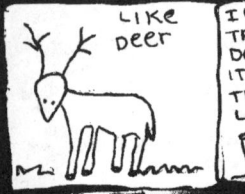

| LIKE DEER | IF A COUGAR IS TRYING TO GET A DEER, RIGHT BEFORE IT CATCHES IT, THE DEER WILL LAY DOWN AND FREEZE | | IT'S HEART BEAT SLOWS ♡ | IT'S BREATH QUIETS ⅂ ⅂ IT'S MUSCLES RIDGID |

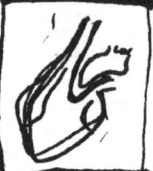

it won't move an inch.

A friend of mine tells me about this. She says "frozen, the soul can go somewhere where it won't be touched. Frozen, maybe the cougar will just pass it by. Frozen, if it does get killed, maybe it doesn't hurt as much."

I laugh, nervous laugh, because do I believe in soul? Plus, it always hurt pretty bad the times I've been assaulted and/or raped while frozen (why didn't I do something? Why didn't they notice? Why did it happen at all?)

My friend says "one of the differences between us and the deer is that once the danger is past, the deer find their family and then they shake and shake, get the trauma out of their bodies, somewhere safe, with the protective family around. Where do we get that release and support?"

"At the punk show?" I say.

"Come on now, really." She says, and of course, it is true. It is not the same. She says "we don't get support and release. We are almost never in a place of safty. The trauma builds in us. We freeze our voices, our bodies. We become frozen inside."

She thinks it is instinct and culture. I think it is systematic oppression and patriarchy. But sometimes now, alone in my room, I shake and I shake and I scream.

frozen inside 2

Maybe we need 100 new words for when our friends or acquaintances or partners assault or rape us. One word to describe, "I let you because I was half asleep and too tired to do anything else." One that's "I was to sick of arguing about it." One for "It's fucked up and scary the way you talk to me. One for "I told you I didn't want to do that." One for, "why didn't you notice I wasn't present anymore." One for, "we had an agreement you would use protection." One for, "you said if I didn't do it you'd leave me. What choice did I have?"

Maybe we need 100 new words to talk about rape and sexual assault and sexual manipulation: words that speak clear about the seriousness of what is being done to our bodies. Or maybe our friends and acquaintances and partners need to have the courage to hear "You raped me, ore "that was assault" (I still barely ever use these words because I know the backlash consequences. I know that no one has the courage to hear their actions defined that way. They don't want to admit they are capable of rape or assault. They don't want to admit that patriarchy exists and that it gives them the God and State granted rights to do these things. They don't want to look at the physical and political nature of their actions. They want to blow it all off. They have a million different reasons for what they did.)

Every time I've tried to talk to someone about sexual stuff that they did to me that I didn't want, their first reaction is to (usually frantically) try to explain it away. They want the story to different than the one I'm telling. They want me to see it through their eyes and absolve them. They say "But I thought," they say, "I never would have," even "No, that's not what happened" (as if their experience was the only one). They try to make me out as crazy. They say I am blaming them for things that are really just stored up from my past.

I am not crazy. I am aware that capitalism and patriarchy and all systems of control depend on the denial of both the oppressor and the oppressed. I know that patriarchy values logic over emotion, and that "too much" emotion, too strong of a response, will label you crazy, and that women especially are considered crazy lot of the time. We are not crazy. What happens to us is real. All the attempts to silence us won't change this reality.

I carry with me a whole history of sexual abuse, and so do most of us. Each sexual act does not exist in a vacuum and I'm sick of people treating it as if it does. I never want to hear the fucking words, "Well, why didn't you stop me?" again. I want to hear, "oh my god, I'm so sorry" and then I want them to ask for my story. I want them to be able to take it instead of asking for pity. If I tell them to fuck off and leave me alone, then I want them to respect that. If it's someone I love, I might want them to hold me so I can cry. If it's someone I hate, I want to be able to punch them without the community saying "dude, that's so fucked up! She hit him!"

I want all of them to say, I believe you. I'm taking this seriously. I hate what I've done and I'm going to change. I'm going to commit myself (or recommit myself) to looking deep inside of myself and changing my behavior and looking at this world and what it's made me into, and it's my responsibility. I'm going to take this seriously. Thank you for having the courage to tell me. I'm going to work as hard as possible to make sure I never do that to anyone ever again."

I want them to say that and feel it and mean it and follow through.

Supporting Someone Who's Reliving Sexual Assault

What I want to talk about might seem overwhelming and scary but it happens sometimes and the more of us who know how to help the better. Many people who have been sexually assaulted develop a condition called Post Traumatic Stress Disorder, PTSD for short. The National Institute of Mental Health defines PTSD as "an anxiety disorder that can develop after exposure to a terrifying event or ordeal in which grave physical harm occurred or was threatened." They cite personal assaults, natural or human caused disasters, accidents, or military combat as experiences that can trigger PTSD. The disorder is characterized by various degrees of re-experiencing the trauma: recurrent memories, nightmares, frightening thoughts, and what I want to discuss here, flashback episodes. Other symptoms are sleep disturbance, emotional numbness, anxiety, irritability, depression, and outbursts of anger.

Though this cluster of symptoms has probably been around as long as people have been hurting each other, it was not diagnosed until men began to exhibit symptoms in great numbers during and following World War I. Before, women were considered by the medical establishment to be the only bearers of physical manifestations of a mental condition; the disorder was then called hysteria and was generally considered a contrivance of attention seeking females. World War I sent home men who had experienced more than their minds could bear. They relived their scenes of war, their bodies shut down; they could not function. Suddenly, doctors decided that this mental state, shell shock they called it, could happen to anyone, not only to members of what they considered the weaker sex. What had previously been viewed the folly of women became a legitimate disorder worthy of attention. This attention unfortunately usually consisted primarily of institutionalization and medication.

However negative the treatment, at least people who suffered from this disorder had a name for it. They could see that the mind sometimes collapses under stress, that this is a normal response to unbearable strain, not a sign of weakness. As the women's movement of the 70's grew, women who began to examine sexual assault and its effects saw the symptoms of PTSD in many women who had been assaulted or had lived in abusive environments. People who wanted to create a supportive framework for dealing with sexual assault developed strategies for helping people who exhibited signs of what they called Rape Trauma Syndrome. These strategies were implemented and taught to volunteers throughout the network of Rape Crisis Centers and Women's Shelters and they still are today.

When I trained at a Rape Crisis Center, we spent part of one short class talking about what to do if a client started to relive an assault. Many of the volunteers expressed concerns that they were not prepared to deal with such an extreme situation. Our advisor explained that it hardly ever happened and she hadn't had to deal with a flashback in all her years at the center.

At least we spent those few minutes on flash backs because within a few weeks, one of my clients showed up at the center fully in the throes of reliving a rape. She had been in an abusive marriage for years, during which time her husband repeatedly raped her. Though she had been on her own for a while and lived in a different town than him, she still had nightmares and felt continually unsafe. I don't remember what triggered her flashback, but it happened while she was driving. Luckily, she was near the Center and could just pull in there. She walked in shaking and staring straight ahead. I led her to the couch as she described her assault as it was happening. She was terrified.

First, I slowly put my arms around her and spoke in a low voice, telling her she was in a safe place. Here is the important part: since the person is not in the present moment, you need to get them someplace safe in their mind. This might sound silly but it works. As they told us to do in training, I told her to picture a safe place and put herself there, a place where no can get her and she feels free from any possible harm. I then asked her to describe the place to me. This gives the person something to do, a task to occupy the mind until the crisis is over. She told me about a boat. I asked a lot of questions about the boat, the area around the boat. No question is too detailed. The person needs to focus on this safe place. After a few minutes of describing her boat, she quit shaking, her heartbeat slowed down, and her eyes saw her immediate surroundings again. She was still upset, but the crisis was over. We talked until she felt okay to leave and I checked on her frequently for the next few days.

The fact is, you may never be around when someone you know relives a trauma. But if you are, remember these few things:

1) Speak in soothing tones.

2) If you touch the person, be gentle as you comfort them, there's a fine line between feeling held and feeling held down.

3) Ask them to picture a safe place and to tell you all about it.

4) Ask a lot of questions so they really have to inhabit the safe place.

5) Once the immediate crisis is over, talk to the person about what happened, what triggered the flashback.

6) Make a plan to stay with your friend or find another person they trust to stay with them if you have to leave.

7) Offer to be available for the person to talk to or spend time with in the immediate future.

8) Remember, these symptoms may get better with time but you will probably need to actively support this person for a long time. They are dealing with a lot and this flashback is just an extreme manifestation of what they think of every day.

9) While therapy is sometimes maligned in our community, it can be very helpful. When someone is dealing with this much mental stress, talking to a trained counselor is probably a good idea. Don't be afraid to suggest this option.

10) Keep up the support, keep checking in.

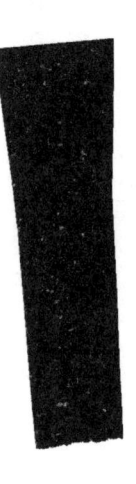

things to do when you are having trouble staying present

BLINK HARD. BLINK AGAIN. DO IT ONCE MORE AS HARD AS YOU CAN.

MAKE TEA. DRINK IT.

CALL A FRIEND.

EAT A SNACK.

JUMP UP AND DOWN WAVING YOUR ARMS.

LIE DOWN ON THE FLOOR; FEEL YOUR BODY CONNECTING WITH IT. KEEP YOUR EYES OPEN. HOW DOES IT FEEL? DESCRIBE IT OUT LOUD TO YOURSELF.

MAKE EYE CONTACT WITH YOUR PET. NOW HOLD IT.

CLAP YOUR HANDS.

BREATHE DEEPLY. KEEP BREATHING. PAY ATTENTION TO YOUR EVERY BREATH.

HOLD A STUFFED ANIMAL, PILLOW, OR YOUR FAVORITE BLANKET.

ALTERNATELY TENSE AND RELAX SOME MUSCLES.

NOW "BLINK" WITH YOUR WHOLE BODY, NOT JUST YOUR EYELIDS.

MOVE YOUR EYES FROM OBJECT TO OBJECT, STOPPING TO FOCUS ON EACH ONE.

WASH YOUR FACE.

GO OUTSIDE FOR SUNSHINE OR FRESH AIR.

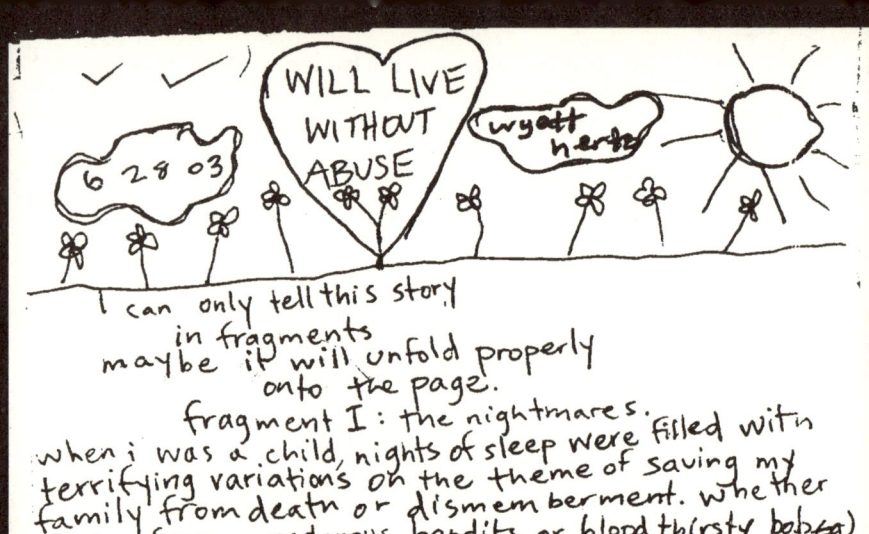

I can only tell this story
in fragments
maybe it will unfold properly
onto the page.

fragment I: the nightmares.
when i was a child, nights of sleep were filled with terrifying variations on the theme of saving my family from death or dismemberment. whether it be from murderous bandits or bloodthirsty bobcats. i was responsible for hiding them away and securing the house. my father was not present in these dreams. i have now realized that the threat to the safety of my loved ones was a representation of he, himself. i failed to save them, going lame as i attempted to reach the last door and laying paralized as screams permeated the house.

fragment II: waking life

am.: some mornings for no logical reason, he would get angry and explode, refuse to let us go to school, and confine us to washing the walls of the house. one day, he became irate about the simple disorder of our bedrooms and thrashed around destroying our belongings, dumping out drawers, knocking things from shelves, and overturning our beds. we were not allowed to leave the house that day.
p.m.: terror strikes after 6. he's home. if we tip toe he won't know we're here. go to sleep. go to sleep. good sleep.

(heart) WILL LIVE WITHOUT ABUSE
6 28 03
wyatt hertz

fragment III: the images

mom in the bathtub, it's empty and he's holding her down by the red handkercheif around her neck i'm standing in the doorway trying to block my brother's view. at the dinner table, he's got my little brother by the neck he slams his little body against the wall 6 feet high against one of grandmother's paintings i hear the glass crack in the frame. he's dragging my sister by her hair, through the gravel driveway. i only remember the belt. i'm confused. i can't remember what he did to me. do they?

fragment IV:

mommie,
   why why why ~~mama~~
why   did   you   stay   with him?
why didn't you leave the first time it happened? why did you let him hurt me? you could not disguise it with sunglasses and makeup. you should not have been struck because there was no meat for lunch. nor i, by you, for letting an ink pen leak on your comforter. i love you. your tender touches soothed me.

the whole picture

how does one deal when dealt this hand in life? alone in the woods and afraid, i was always ~~struck~~ in pain people i loved pulled me towards them, and as i was enjoying the closeness, shoved me away. becoming accustomed to this treatment, i began to expect it from anyone involved with me personally. trust meant nothing to me.

 i'm trying to get better, to rid myself of these demons they will kill me if i let them. i want love, and, to love, without hurt. i will cure myself and i won't be mad anymore. i won't take any hush money because i needed to let someone know.

> have love   will live   ♡♡

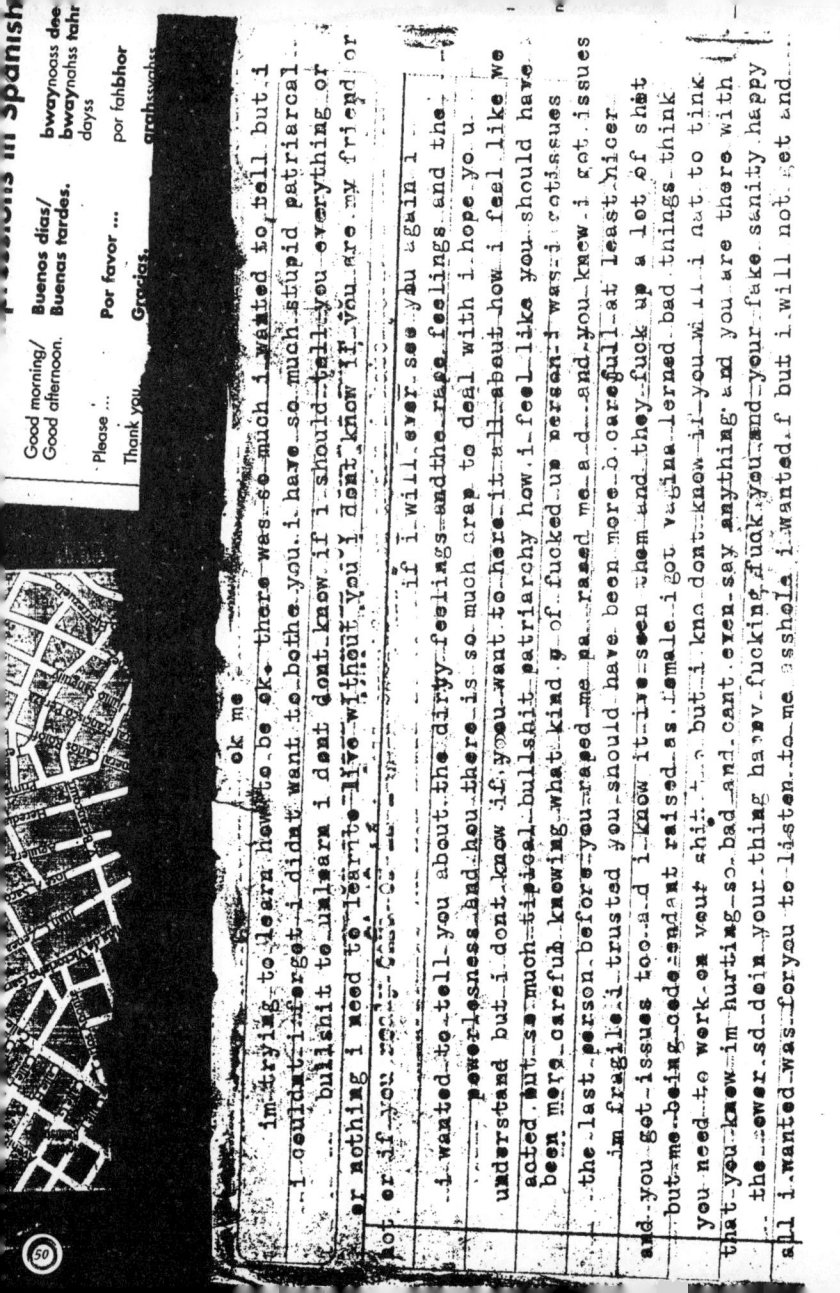

Good morning/ Good afternoon.	Buenos días/ Buenos tardes.	bwaynoass dee-ass/ bwaynahss tahr-dayss
Please ...	Por favor ...	por fahbhor
Thank you.	Gracias.	grahssyahss

ok me

im trying to learn how to be ok. there was so much i wanted to tell but i
i couldnt i forget i didnt want to bothe you. i have so much stupid patriarcal
bullshit to unlearn i dont dont know if i should tell you everything or
or nothing i need to learn to live without you. i dont know if you are my friend or
not or if you are... if i will ever see you again i
i wanted to tell you about the dirty feelings and the rage feelings and the
powerlesness bad how there is so much crap to deal with i hope you u
understand but i dont know if you want to here it all about how i feel like we
acted but so much tipical bullshit patriarchy how i feel like you should have
been more careful knowing what kind g of fucked up person i was i got issues
the last person before you raped me a and you know i got issues
im fragile i trusted you should have been more o carefull at least nicer
and you got issues too a d i know it it i ve seen them and they fuck up a lot of shit
but me being codependant raised as femal e i got vagina lerned bad things think
you need to work on your shit and but i kno dont know if you wi ll i nat to tink
that you know im hurting so bad and cant even say anything and you are there with
the ower sd dein your thing ha rev fucking fuck you and your fake sanity happy
all i wanted was for you to listen to me asshole i wanted f but i will not get and

im having treuble getting ever it i get t o much stupid issues coming up and
and your face haunts me in the f middle of them and i hate you forit ill even though
        itws only sme your fault i hated you and your ability to not care and just
do stuff and fuck people and be ok i hate being fucked up i thought for a second
that im met out im thinking i might realy be ok i might recly be fucked up for the
rest of my life ad and that scares me i dont like it at all i want to be happy i dont
know how to right noward you get the last laugh assholl all of t em get lthe last
lauph cuz we are th ones fucked up for the rest of ourfucking lives ad we cant even
have "partners" who use t at word to fuckin be sensitive thy only pretend you only
waned in my pants and andw em you got in you were done fuck you congradulations you
you get the burden of being the first one to fuck mesince ive been raped and you got
to leave it and i dont fuck you asshole and you didnt efen do it nicly s o dont ever
tell me you love me i hate you i ha te you for not being considerate of my heart
and not knowing how to b e
how to be a friend when i tll you i need a friend you say you are a my friend
and then you cant even be there for me cuz you still havent learned how.

For my father...

By jake holloway

Last time I saw my father, he sat across from me at dinner and told me about the face of the monster that would appear to him out of nowhere when he tried to sleep at night. It was the horrible, half-eaten face of a dog, all fangs and teeth and ripped flesh. It would loom over him in the dark.

My father's stories. They would cling to me like tiny shards of glass. He would toss them at me over breakfast. Sweep them under my feet on the back porch. Offer them up in our crowded family car, and I would choke on tobacco smoke and the burden of too many splintered memories swallowed whole.

He stopped drinking when I was eleven. When you stop drinking, there are one or two years of bliss. Effortless life. The exhilaration of clear vision and shaky nervous fingers. They call this the honeymoon period. And then all at once, the darkness melts away and all those terrible stories you tried to obscure blossom into sharp and distinct forms, gleaming teeth and broken edges.

This is when the memories of my grandmother began to surface.

I don't know details really.

I don't want to.

When her second husband died, she took my father into her bedroom, and told him that he was the man of the house.

I am sitting in the back seat of the car. I only want to hear the music on the radio.

My grandmother's eyes are small and glowing like glass beads. She is young for her age. Her ankles are thin and fragile like mine. She is still very much alive despite her catheter and sunken cheeks. I wait patiently by the bed. I feed her jello while my father paces the halls. She is dripping like a wilted flower. She reveals herself-all folded flesh and blue veins, her colostomy bag spilling along the white linoleum. I watch her struggle, humiliated and stunned by her own fading life.

I watch my father and his boyish terror.

I watch my own eyes in the mirror of the house I grew up in. I look for pieces of her shimmering in my quivering lips and my broken gaze.

I don't want this woman to exist inside my skin, dendrites tracing paths forged by her

I don't want to know.

My father was raped on Neptune Beach. He'd been looking for perfect conk shells without missing pieces.

Some man asked my father if he wanted to go on a ride.

He took my father to a hotel room and held a blade to his throat.

My father lived with a man once, a composer named Jonathon. They lived together for 10 years. This was before he met my mother.

My father was a young, promising actor. He and Jonathon drank together and wrote songs. Brilliant songs.

This man feared fame more than life. He locked himself in a cheap hotel the night his play made it onto Broadway.

He died recently. He'd been living in a one-bedroom apartment in a housing project in South Georgia. He was studying the Roman Empire and the music of Croatia.

My father always had ways of escaping, even when he was small. He would run out to the trapeze in the backyard. He would swing skyward and sail above barns and red clay, chicken bones, threadbare tires, shotgun shells, bits of china gleaming under a godlike southern sun. He would swing up and up and up

He would go to the movies on Saturdays and disappear into silvery California moonlight, floor length satin gowns; swelling violins. Romance and cowboys and men in velvet waistcoats. Marilyn Monroe! My father knew he could save her from the pills and the pain of stardom. He wrote her letters and her press agent sent him an autographed photo that he kept under his pillow.

Oh god, these stories pile up around my brittle ankles, sink into my skin.

There was the stark, swollen grip of the drunk who married his mother. He would chase them outside in the dead of night with a rifle in his hand, firing shots that sank into the flaccid soil of the cotton fields. He would read my father's fortune in coffee grounds. He would toss empty bottles at the wall.

And one day he draped his hands over my father's shoulders and his hands were like buckets of moonshine, heavy and damp and spilling over the edge. And this man, this man who wandered through the house like a pixilated beast, who tossed china out of doorways and shattered windows, this man looked deep into my fathers already frantic eyes and said, "You are my son."

I have always known that I am my father's daughter. I can tell by the way I twist little pieces of paper into spirals between my fingers. I can tell by the way darkness wraps around my brain like a raincoat. I can hear his nervous laugh rattling in my rib cage. We both have trouble breathing while we sleep.

My veins are swollen and heavy with thick blood. I am carrying memories that are not mine. My cells are saturated with secrets. I am listening to stories whispered across the table, through the closed door, over the back seat.

I don't want to know.
I don't want to know.
I only want to hear the music on the radio.

Awkwardly I stumbled.

When I was a boy of 16 I fell in love. I fell for a girl who had a long story. She'd gotten hooked on dope young and wound up living through a lot of shit that many people do but no one should have to.

She loved me, but the scars from her past bulged tender. I'd been lucky. At that age, I didn;t know the feel of sexual abuse. I didn;t know what it felt like to sell the use of my body.

Awkwardly I stumbled. I hated my body for reminding her of people who had violated hers. I hated myself because I was certain that every time she cried when we were together, it was something I'd done. My narcissism and the self-concious natureoof my uncertainty in something new made me try to make it right. I wanted to fix it, fix her, erase the parts of the world that caused her pain.

I was lucky that she gave enough of a shit about me to teach me. She taught me that there were no words that could take away the past. Life is written in pen.

I learned to stop apologizing out of fear of her emotions. To just hold her because sometime she needed to cry, because some people take not of anniversaries that are not happy.

We talked and talked. She told me about what it was like in her head and I ceased to pity her but marvel at her instead. Lifehad hurt her but she had healed stronger. I was in awe of the courage that it took for her to laugh. The courage it took for her to trust. She taught me what it it meant to be a survivor, to actively survive something not once but daily. She taught me more than I could ever put in to words. I just want to thank her and every other teacher. Please keep teaching, you never know when you're teaching someone more than how to empathize but something that will help them stay alive too.

Keep laughing, keep dancing, you don't always know how much your strength inspires. Many superheros have torn capes, many angels have had scared wings.

One girlfriend I had, her previous boyfriend used to beat
her up. I was clueless, cruel, cold-hearted and eighteen.
I think she loved me because I didn't hit her. I wasn't
very kind otherwise.
The next girlfriend I had told me she wasn't into blowjobs
because she used to have to give them to her uncle. We
often had sex with our clothes on. The last six months of
our relationship we had sex twice. I didn't know how to
process the information about her and her uncle. Somehow I
knew it wasn't unusual, and I guess having clear parameters
(no blowjobs) made it an easy thing for me to avoid, and
still feel like I was doing alright by her.
A few years later I got very drunk at a house show. I ran
into a friend there and she gave me a ride back to her house.
We made out and then she undressed me and we had sex. I
didn't want to, but I was drunk and something said as a
guy I shouldn't feel uncomfortable. My body was reacting,
but I felt terrible and something in my head told me it was
weak to say no.
The next day we went to an amusement park and sat on a
bench. I threw up in the garbage can repeatedly. She took
me home. I was very hungover, disgusted with myself and
her. I knew it wasn't the biggest thing— so minor compared
to what every woman I'd had a relationship with had experienced. I was mad at her for doing that, for not asking.
I was mad at myself for getting into that situation with
an old friend. I kept telling myself it wasn't that big
a deal, but I left town without telling anyone for two weeks.

◆

It was a awhile before I had any kind of sexual contact with
anyone again.
With the next girlfriend, things went very slow.
When I think about what it might mean to be a good partner
to someone, I think of her. The way she talked about her
own expierences and talked to me about mine. "Is this OK?"
"Why does this feel weird?" I didn't tell her at first
but she kept asking in a way that was gentle and patient.
It seemed seamless.
I still don't get it, but I'm more careful then I used to
be, I'm more aware. I'm used to being seen as a good guy,
or (lord forbid) a sensitive guy, but I know that in reality
it hasn't added up to shit because other people's abuse was
something I had to negotiate. I never went out of my way to
understand it or deal with it until my own boundaries were
crossed in such a minor way.

i didn't realize the complexities of denial. i never knew that it could possess layers upon layers of it's own truth. i didn't comprehend that denial could have it's own purpose beyond what i could understand. mostly, i didn't know that denial was my protection.

i'm not even talking about the denial that saved me as a child: all families are like mine, my mom loves me, things aren't so bad, things could be worse.

no, i'm talking about the denial i've had in my healing process. alot of it was the same mantras as before, but in a different context: piece of cake, i can get over this standing on my head. it wasn't so horrible, i'm still alive. it wasn't so horrible, i'm not in an institution. it wasn't so bad, i haven't tried to kill myself in years. i'm making such a big deal out of nothing. after all, everyone gets depressed. everyone is suicidal.

so why do i say denial was a good thing? because it saved me from having to take on the full weight of what has happened to me all at once.

denial

i still have my moments of denial, and maybe i will for the rest of my life. for the most part it's gone. at it's height, i couldn't wish it away fast enough. i just wanted to be sure, i wanted to believe my memories 150% without a doubt. now that i do, i am often plagued by something more difficult to deal with than denial. sadness. for if i believe fully in the memories i have uncovered, then i must believe those memories are true and real. and if i believe they are true, then i must accept that they really happened to me.

sadness feels weird. depression, i know like the back of my hand. depression comes in big waves, and it's a struggle just to get out of bed. eventually, it ends. sadness is different. it comes and goes. i never see it until it's right in front of me. sleep won't make it go away, there is no "anti-sadness" medication on the market. it's not debilitating, it's just an all-body experience, like a sigh from the bottom of me that just keeps coming out. i never know when i'll get to take in another breath.

healing, like denial, is multi-layered. it's important to have tunnel vision, to constantly remember that all of this is leading toward a brighter place. the thing is, healing doesn't always feel like healing, sometimes it just hurts. in those moments, looking for the better place seems like denial itself. maybe it is, and maybe that's why it works.

Lists

Write down everything you can think of that is beautiful, that makes you feel alive, or that you simply *like*. It's so easy for people like us to forget these things when we're in our lows and reconnecting to them, even by name, helps us to bring them back into our lives. Here are a few of the things on my list: moments of total silence on a city street; freshly opened lilacs; the smell of old books; drinking water when I'm really thirsty; cobalt blue glass; really good letters; the color of my skin under a full moon; wind; listening to In Utero by Nirvana; the color green, deep, deep green; cool velvet on my ears and cheeks; the smell of sheep; fresh, clean socks. This is the comfort food of my life and I had more or less forgotten about it, all of it, until I wrote it all down.

In addition to the list of things to live for is a list of actions that you know will help to pull you out of your shit if you're in a bad way. Examples could be anything from taking a walk around your neighborhood to eating a good meal to spending time with your dog. Give copies of this list to your close friends so they have some idea of how to help you when you're not okay. Also a good tool to give to those trusted allies is a list of warning signs that you're sinking into a bad place. The signs could be subtle, like circles around your eyes from lack of sleep, or they could be blatant, such as not leaving your bedroom for three days. Even if these things seem obvious to you, it's important that you identify them to you friends so they know to come to your aid quickly, when the warning signs first start to appear.

There is one more list that you cannot do without and this is a list of the people you will contact when you are feeling fucked up or are in the depths of some kind of crisis. Do this when you're in a relatively level headspace because if you try to do it when a panic is asphyxiating you or when you're paralyzed by depression you will have a very hard time thinking of anyone and this will make you feel ten times worse. Keep this list somewhere accessible, laminate it with packing tape and stick it to your phone or to your bathroom mirror or make a few copies of it in case you lose one. Even if it doesn't sound important now, it will be. Believe me.

Crisis

Okay, this is the most appropriate method I can think of to deal with a panic attack-type situation. It is what I wish someone had told me when I was collapsing under the weight of fear and despair.

1) Breathe. Put your right hand on your belly and breathe into it deeply, feeling it expand. Now exhale for *twice as long* as your inhalation, you can count seconds if you want to. This will bring your heart rate to a steady pace and will keep your system from getting overloaded with oxygen, now you won't pass out.
Repeat this process. Stay conscious of your breathing.
Remember this: **If you're still breathing you are still alive.**

2) If you are not home right now, if you are at a show or a restaurant or are traveling and are in common space at a stranger's house, quietly leave the room. When there are lots of people around me and I feel the way you're feeling, it tends to make it worse. If you're with a friend, ask them to come with you. If you're alone, it's still okay, you can still be safe. Go out to the yard or an empty room or the bathroom, somewhere you won't attract a lot of attention and where you are not in physical danger.
Don't move very far. Walk slowly and don't talk to any cops.

3) Now, come back to your body. You might not be able to feel your limbs right now, maybe not your skin either and this is okay. It's a reasonable response to fear, but returning awareness to your body will do a lot to make you feel safe. If you have someone you trust close by, ask them to hold you, very gently. Focus on their arms supporting you, keeping you safe. If you're alone, wrap your own arms around you.
Sit down somewhere, a soft place if you can find one, and slowly, gently, rock back and forth.
Your body remembers this from when you were a baby and it will comfort you now just like it did then.
Keep breathing, each exhale twice as long as the inhale.
If you are still dissociating (retreating from your body) close your eyes and imagine you are filling yourself back up again. Imagine a warm, white light pouring into your feet and filling you up…moving through your legs…up your torso…into your shoulders (*keep breathing*)…down your arms and into your hands…up your neck…into your face…all the way up to the top of your head. Now you are full.
Rock gently back and forth until the rhythm naturally slows itself, until you are still and safe.
Keep breathing, each exhale twice as long as the inhale.

4) If you're alone and are still nowhere near okay, find your list of people to call when you feel like this.
If they are not answering, call the next person and then the next one. Go all the way down the list, and back up to the top if necessary, until you reach someone. Tell them exactly what's going on with you.

5) **Don't fight it.** I cannot stress enough that the only way to get through difficult feelings is to *let yourself feel them*. Trying desperately to hold at bay everything raging inside you, will only intensify the storm. You must *move through* these feelings. Don't deny the experience, see it for what it is. Name it: "I feel really scared right now," "I feel like the walls are closing in on me," "I feel like I'm sinking."
And just hang out with it. Don't let it consume you, don't let it be everything that you are. Recognize it for what it is, a feeling, and then let it move through you. Soften into it and be with it and it will pass through ten times more quickly and cleanly than if you clench onto it.

59

If You Are Not the One Falling Apart

As a supporter, the most vital tool available to you is empathy. I know how hard it is for you, your task is to realize how hard it is for him. Try to bring yourself back to a time when you were struggling like your friend is struggling now. Remember how it feels to need support. You will need patience, you will need a clear idea of what you can and cannot do and you must communicate this to your friend.

It can get really hard and really scary; there will be times when you don't know what to do or if there is *anything* you can do to help this person you care for so much. *Do your support work as a team.* It is the best way to preserve your own mental health and relieves a ton of pressure. You get a break from the whirlwind as well as time for your personal self care. Meet together with the other supporters and check in with one another. Fill each other in on how the process is going and what needs to change. It really does help to be organized about this.

Some responsibilities of supporters might include: Really basic survival stuff like getting your friend to eat, go outside, and get plenty of sleep; a person who is falling apart in a serious way can't be expected to have healthy habits of any kind. And because healthy habits are part of what will help him get through this, you might have to make them happen for him, at least in the beginning. Use the cards your friend made with advice on how to pull him out of his shit. You may need to take initiative in getting your friend to see his counselor or go to yoga class. If he is on medication, get him to take his drugs at regular times each day and if he runs out you may need to make an appointment with a psychiatrist for him. Network with his family or a really old friend who's known him for years and find out how they've dealt with situations like this in the past.

It is *not* appropriate for you to try to fix your friend, don't take away his agency like that. He has to "fix" himself, that's why he's falling apart in the first place. As a supporter it is your job to create a safe environment for your friend to experience what he needs to, not to make his problems go away.

The most important thing is that you stay out of judgment. You may find you're carrying more weight than you think you deserve but you have to remind yourself of your love for this person, of everything he gives you when he is well enough to give. This is your friend. The part you play in his well being should be a gift you give, not a burden you shoulder. Stay open and be honest, with yourself and with your friend, about your own needs and limits. Keep the lines of communication open, especially if you're nearing the end of your rope, and have empathy, no matter how hard it gets. Treat your friend as you would treat any fragile and vulnerable creature: very gently, with kindness and great care.

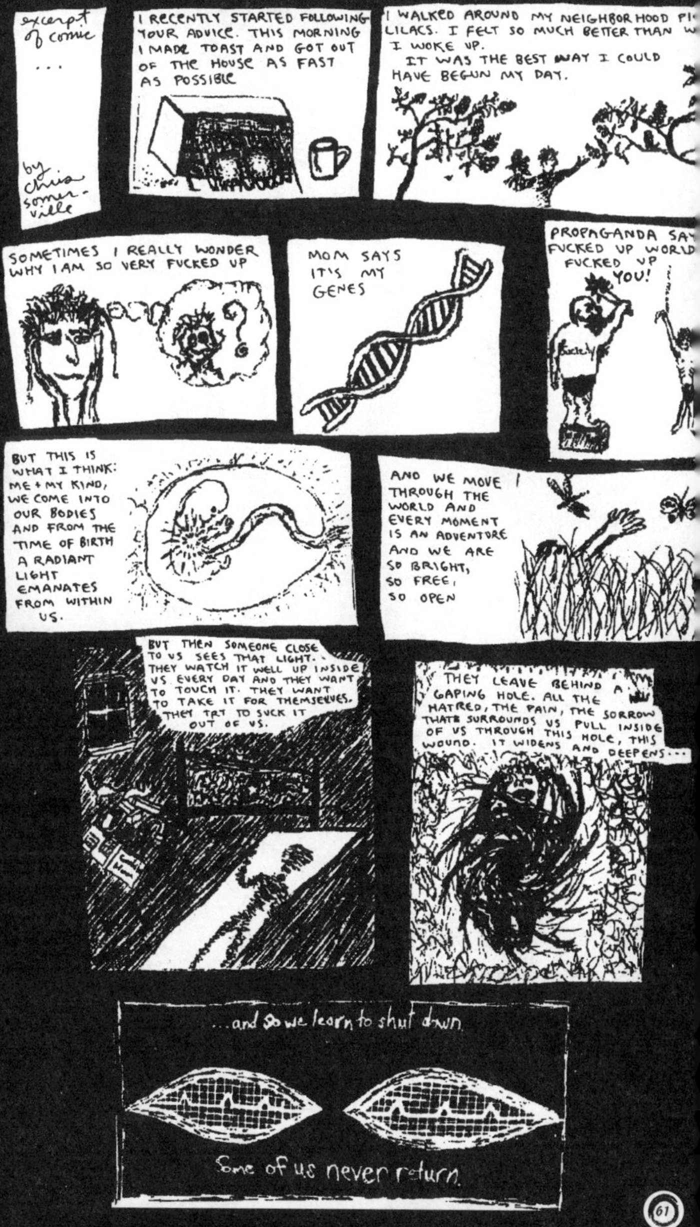

excerpt of comic...

by chris somer- ville

I RECENTLY STARTED FOLLOWING YOUR ADVICE. THIS MORNING I MADE TOAST AND GOT OUT OF THE HOUSE AS FAST AS POSSIBLE

I WALKED AROUND MY NEIGHBORHOOD PI[CKING] LILACS. I FELT SO MUCH BETTER THAN W[HEN] I WOKE UP.
IT WAS THE BEST WAY I COULD HAVE BEGUN MY DAY.

SOMETIMES I REALLY WONDER WHY I AM SO VERY FUCKED UP

MOM SAYS IT'S MY GENES

PROPAGANDA SAY[S] FUCKED UP WORLD FUCKED UP YOU!

BUT THIS IS WHAT I THINK: ME & MY KIND, WE COME INTO OUR BODIES AND FROM THE TIME OF BIRTH A RADIANT LIGHT EMANATES FROM WITHIN US.

AND WE MOVE THROUGH THE WORLD AND EVERY MOMENT IS AN ADVENTURE AND WE ARE SO BRIGHT, SO FREE, SO OPEN

BUT THEN SOMEONE CLOSE TO US SEES THAT LIGHT. THEY WATCH IT WELL UP INSIDE US EVERY DAY AND THEY WANT TO TOUCH IT. THEY WANT TO TAKE IT FOR THEMSELVES. THEY TRY TO SUCK IT OUT OF US.

THEY LEAVE BEHIND A GAPING HOLE. ALL THE HATRED, THE PAIN, THE SORROW THAT SURROUNDS US PULL INSIDE OF US THROUGH THIS HOLE, THIS WOUND. IT WIDENS AND DEEPENS...

...and so we learn to shut down.

Some of us never return.

BUT DENYING THE EXISTANCE OF OUR WOUNDS IS NOT THE ANSWER

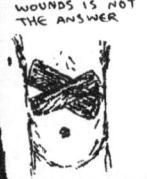

WE HAVE TO REMAIN OPEN ENOUGH TO SEE ALL THOSE THINGS THAT MOST PEOPLE CAN'T SEE

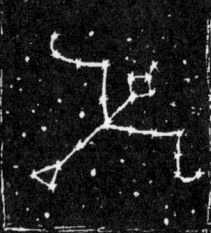

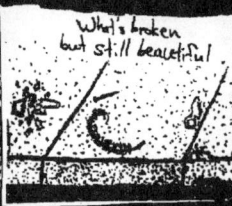

What's broken but still beautiful

SOMEONE TOLD ME ONCE THAT THE VERY BEST THERAPY IS DOING THE THINGS YOU FEEL MOST PASSIONATE ABOUT AS MUCH AS YOU CAN

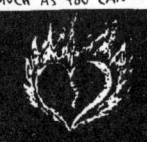

LITTLE THINGS THAT MEAN A LOT.

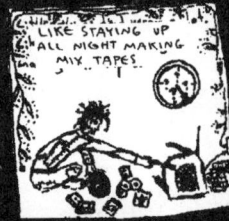

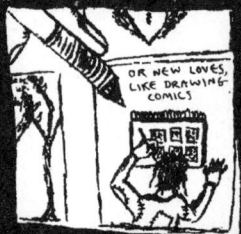

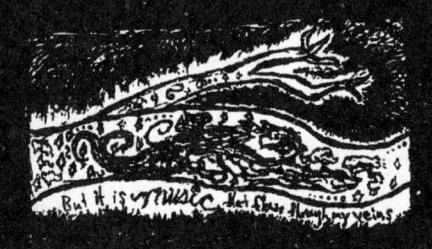

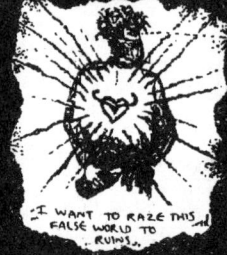

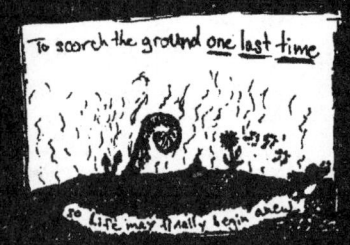

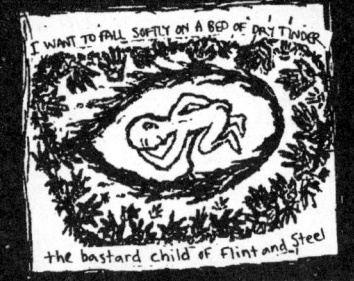

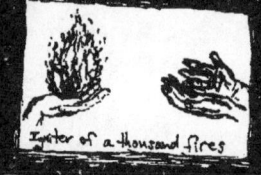

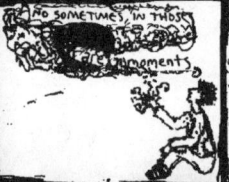

LIKE STAYING UP ALL NIGHT MAKING MIX TAPES

OR NEW LOVES, LIKE DRAWING COMICS

But it is music that flows through my veins

...I WANT TO RAZE THIS FALSE WORLD TO RUINS...

To scorch the ground one last time

so life may finally begin anew

I WANT TO FALL SOFTLY ON A BED OF DRY TINDER

the bastard child of Flint and Steel

Igniter of a thousand fires

No sometimes, in those fragments

when the fog clears

when I can finally HEAR myself again

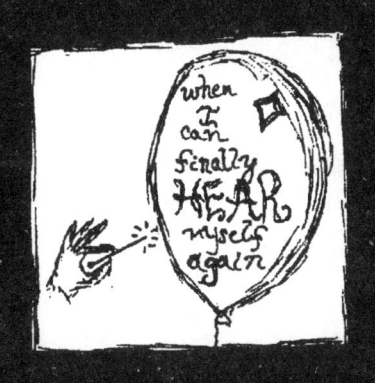

I go inside
And I listen
And I KNOW

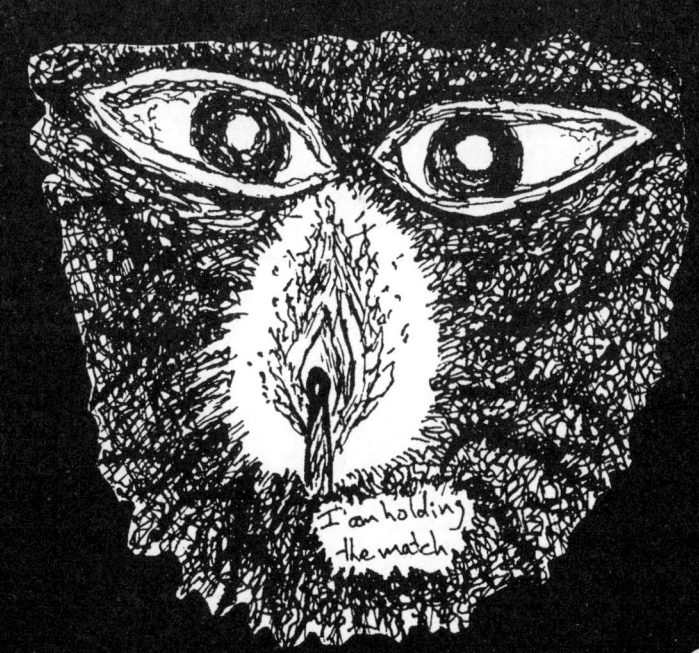

I am holding the match

Credits and Resources

♥ there were alot of people who wanted to remain anonomous - and some who I wasn't sure of and so I put them anonomous too. I wrote a few things anonomously as well.

THANKS TO EVERYONE! THERE WERE MANY OTHER LETTERS + STORIES THAT DESERVE TO BE HEARD! I COULDN'T FIT IT ALL IN + I'M SORRY.

COVER - **CRISTY ROAD** - check out her zine GREEN ZINE available through MICROCOSM

FLY did the comic I excerpted on p.11. She does a regular comic in SLUG + LETTUCE and has a book out called PEOPS and some zines.

ME - I did LISTENING p 8+9 and FROZEN INSIDE p 39-42 also reprinted from S+L

CHRIS SOMERVILLE - wrote "safe sex for survivors" p 15-21 I excerpted parts of "HEALING, MENTAL HEALTH + SELF CARE" which I wish everyone could read all of - 509 GARRISON ST. NE. OLY WA 98506 also he did the comic p.61-63

ANANDI - wrote p.22-25 for MRR and let me reprint it here

JANET - wrote p.34-37 and also p.43-46. She writes zines sometimes one called ROCKET QUEEN

CIBOLA - is a zine I reprinted p.47 and denial p.57

WYATT HERTZ wrote p.48+49

JAKE HALLOWAY p.52-54

and the back cover is reprinted from TYPHOID MARY

BOOKS: THE COURAGE TO HEAL + ALLIES IN HEALING
INVISIBLE GIRLS: THE TRUTH ABOUT SEXUAL ABUSE
a book for teen girls young women
and everyone who cares about them
SURVIVORS GUIDE TO SEX
TRAUMA AND RECOVERY